Lea Maria Franceschi Dallanora
Fabio Jose Dallanora
Bruna Eliza De Dea

Implementation and regularization of the human teeth biobank

Lea Maria Franceschi Dallanora
Fabio Jose Dallanora
Bruna Eliza De Dea

Implementation and regularization of the human teeth biobank

ScienciaScripts

Imprint

Any brand names and product names mentioned in this book are subject to trademark, brand or patent protection and are trademarks or registered trademarks of their respective holders. The use of brand names, product names, common names, trade names, product descriptions etc. even without a particular marking in this work is in no way to be construed to mean that such names may be regarded as unrestricted in respect of trademark and brand protection legislation and could thus be used by anyone.

Cover image: www.ingimage.com

This book is a translation from the original published under ISBN 978-613-9-61704-3.

Publisher:
Sciencia Scripts
is a trademark of
Dodo Books Indian Ocean Ltd. and OmniScriptum S.R.L publishing group

120 High Road, East Finchley, London, N2 9ED, United Kingdom
Str. Armeneasca 28/1, office 1, Chisinau MD-2012, Republic of Moldova, Europe
Printed at: see last page
ISBN: 978-620-7-89821-3

Table of contents:

SUMMARY

Human tooth biobanks are considered an important scientific tool and are increasingly present in Brazilian dental courses. In the Dentistry course at Unoesc, the BDH began on March 17, 2011. Its purpose was to organize and facilitate the collection, storage and allocation of teeth, formalizing their origin and destination and creating ideal conditions for the use of these organs. Thus, this work seeks to demonstrate how the implementation of the BDH at Unoesc took place, from the physical adequacy project, structure for collection, storage and granting, document organization, functionality and bureaucratic facts to the start of its activities and its regulation with CONEP.

Keywords: Human tooth banks. Biobanks. Structured, Organized and Administered.

Chapter 1

1. INTRODUCTION

Human tooth banks, or biobanks as they are known today, are non-profit institutions that must be linked to a college, university or other institution, with the purpose of meeting academic needs by providing human teeth for research or teaching activities (IMPARATO, 2003). Brazil's System of Research Ethics Committees and National Research Ethics Commission (CEP/CONEP) uses the definition of biobank for organized collections of human biological material and associated information, collected and stored for research purposes, complying with pre-defined technical, ethical and operational regulations or standards, under institutional responsibility and under the management of the researcher, without commercial purposes, according to Resolution No. 441, of May 12, 2011, which provides guidelines for the ethical analysis of research projects involving the storage of human biological material or the use of material stored in previous research (BRASIL, CS 2016).

The creation of Human Tooth Banks (HDB) in higher education institutions in Brazil began around the year 2000, with the aim of minimizing the illegal trade in dental structures, as well as developing the perception of students and professionals in the field of Dentistry about Biosafety, legal issues and discussions on Bioethics (PEREIRA, 2012).

Human teeth are used in the pre-clinical laboratory activities of academics, for in vitro research for undergraduate and postgraduate course completion work, because the ethics and research committees require that the origin of the teeth used in the projects be detailed for approval (NASSIF et al, 2003).

Some time ago, human teeth were not given their due value by researchers, teachers or students who used indiscriminate amounts of human teeth in their work, disregarding the ethical and legal aspects involved in their use. It is essential that teeth are used rationally to avoid some of the practices still found today (VANZELLI et al., 2003).

The existence of an institution concerned with the dental organ is justified by legal, bioethical, cultural and social reasons (NASSIF et al., 2003). Thus, the Biobank of human teeth is organized to facilitate the granting, storage and loan of teeth, taking care of their origin, which must have the consent of the consenting party, as well as their destination, creating ideal conditions for the use of these organs in accordance with CNS Resolution No.^{0} 441 of 2011 and MS Ordinance No. 2.201 of 2011, which regulate the activity of Biobanks of biological material for research purposes.

In this context, teeth are now considered human organs and their indiscriminate use is considered illegal. At the same time, National Health Council Resolution^{0} 196/96 was issued, which concerns the storage and use of human biological material for research purposes (BRASIL, 1997; 2001,2011).

The Human Teeth Bank at UNOESC was structured in accordance with research project° 1149/09, process 1255/10 and resolution° 01/CG/11, respecting the institution's statutes. It has its own internal regulations, a physical space that is properly equipped for disinfecting and storing dental elements in accordance with university policy and the economic reality of the region in which it is located. The BDH, which began its existence and organization in March 2011, now has a collection of around 14,000 teeth, which were collected from various sources, including researchers, professors, private clinics and health clinics in the municipality where the BDH is based and in neighbouring municipalities (ZANATTA, 2014). Subsequently, Resolution No.° 441 of 2011 was created, which standardized and regulated the operation of Human Tooth Biobanks in the country, as well as Resolution No.^{0} 466 of 2012, which aims to organize research involving human biological material, this being a complement to Resolution No. 196/96 (BRASIL, 1996).

This project aims to regulate UNOESC's human teeth bank as a biobank with CONEP, in order to meet the need for human teeth in research by dental academics and postgraduates, which is currently documented in accordance with the norms of Resolution No. 466 of 2012.

CHAPTER 2

2. OBJECTIVES

2.1 GENERAL OBJECTIVE

Regulate with CONEP the Biobank of the University of Western Santa Catarina.

2.1.1 Specific objectives

* Regulate UNOESC's human teeth bank as a Biobank with CONEP, in order to continue research with human teeth from this establishment's collection.
* To meet the research needs of students and professors, inherent to the use of human teeth in their research projects.
* To lend the teeth available in the Human Teeth Biobank to undergraduates, postgraduates and researchers in general to enable the development of scientific research.
* Handle the tooth given to the Tooth Biobank correctly during its storage process, respecting biosafety regulations.

CHAPTER 3

3. LITERATURE REVIEW

As of February 4, 1997, law no.[0] 9.434, the use of human organs or tissues without proven origin is considered a crime. Dental organs are routinely used in university dentistry courses and are indispensable for both teaching and research (PINTO et al., 2009).

The Human Teeth Biobank at the University of Sao Paulo's School of Dentistry is one of the first in the country, having been created over 20 years ago, and is considered a benchmark in terms of the creation and development of a HDB. Also noteworthy is the BDH at the School of Dentistry at the Federal University of Ribeirao Preto, which has been operating since 2002 and meets the demand for teeth for undergraduate, postgraduate and research activities (PEREIRA, 2012a).

Currently, the CEP does not approve research using human teeth whose origin has not been proven or legalized. Undergraduate professors have also become aware of the issue and today ask for a smaller number of teeth for practical activities and, when possible, replace human teeth with artificial ones, usually made of acrylic resin. In higher education institutions that don't have a BDH, only prefabricated teeth can be used, the main limitation of which is that they don't fully reproduce the texture and hardness of a human tooth, thus compromising student learning (MELO, 2005; COSTA, 2007). The only problem is that artificial teeth are very expensive (NASSIF et al., 2003).

The BDH is of the utmost importance in guiding and publicizing the ethical and legal use of dental elements, seeking to curb their illegal trade. It also seeks to develop the perception of teachers and researchers in relation to the ways in which used teeth are collected, sterilized, biosecured, stored, loaned and registered, in accordance with the laws in force in the country (MELO, 2005; COSTA, 2007; MAGGIONI, 2010; PEREIRA, 2012).

Therefore, the implementation of a Human Tooth Bank (HDB) in university dentistry courses is of the utmost importance, so that the teeth used by students and professionals have a proven origin, since all the teeth stored in the HDB must have the permission of their guardian (PINTO et al., 2009).

The scientific output available in this area is quite scarce and often the implementation of HDBs occurs on the back of isolated initiatives, thanks to the exchange of information between institutions that have lived through the experience and the difficulties of implementing the HDB itself (MORREIRA, et al., 2009).

3.1 THE STRUCTURE OF TOOTH BIOBANKS

Nassif et al. (2003) argue that, "[...] the difference between the BDH and a 'collection of teeth' is the more careful organization and its broad functionality. As such, the BDH should provide teeth for any and all research to be carried out at the faculty, as well as providing teeth for pre-clinical laboratory training for academics." It is therefore of the utmost importance to strictly control the BDH's internal procedures, which include sorting out the stock of teeth, registering and filing the records of donors and/or beneficiaries.

The creation of a tooth biobank requires an adequate infrastructure, the acquisition of proper equipment, the hiring of specialized technical and auxiliary personnel, as well as the establishment of proper routines that guide all the stages relating to collection, retrieval, classification, processing, quality control, distribution and records. All these requirements imply that a project must be submitted to the institute's board of directors for approval. Secondly, a statute or regulation must be drawn up and approved at a general meeting, which must then be registered with a legal entity registry office (FERREIRA et at., 2003).

Nassif et al. (2003), points out that:

> A laboratory and a support room are needed to carry out the BDH tests. The laboratory must be built in accordance with current health surveillance standards. The equipment needed is related to the selection, cleaning and storage of teeth, such as refrigerators for storing teeth, benches for selecting and cleaning teeth, sinks, cupboards, personal biosafety materials, disinfectant solutions, ultrasound, instruments, laboratory glassware, among other materials. For administration, it is advisable to have an adjoining room with a microcomputer, filing cabinet, fax, telephone, tables, cupboards and other necessary office supplies.

In order to set up a BDH, it must be linked to an educational institution, which means that dental schools are preferred. The rules of the BDH follow the definitions proposed by the board, and it must have a coordinator who is preferably a qualified teacher. This person will be the BDH's representative at meetings or councils, as well as suggesting a team to manage the BDH and taking responsibility for it. The BDH's statutes will be defined by internal regulations, based on the objectives of the BDH. Each member will have a specific role in a group, in which graduate students will also participate (NASSIF et al., 2003).

With its own organization and functionality, the BDH functions as an organ bank, keeping a collection of teeth preserved in conditions that allow them to be used in research and pre-clinical laboratory training in undergraduate courses. The author also points out that tooth banks are not simple "warehouses" of teeth often found in health services or teaching institutions themselves (PINTO et al., 2003).

Ferreira et al. (2003), consider the implementation of BDH in educational institutions to be an irreversible and fundamental process, precisely because they promote the use of the dental organ in an ethical manner.

3.2 FROM THE ORGANIZED

Teeth, as part of the human body, can be used for research, academic studies and restorative treatment. Thus, through the operation of a tooth biobank, which is similar to an organ bank, it becomes necessary for the consenting party to use their teeth, as well as the recipient to receive these teeth to be used as a biological restoration in the case of oral rehabilitation (GARBIN, 2008).

According to Ferreira et al. (2003),

> Two important documents to put in place are the Free and Informed Consent and the Donation Agreement. Care should be taken to obtain a legal opinion on the legality and value of the texts. These documents are compulsory, issued in two copies, one of which accompanies the donated organ from the collection center to the tooth bank, where it will be archived, and the other must be given to the donor. An important aspect is that the Informed Consent form should be explanatory and contain all the information about the disease

and its consequences, as well as the various forms of treatment that are possible. The patient must declare that they are aware of the whole process. In cases of legal impediments, such as mentally handicapped patients, the legal guardian must sign the document.

The use of extracted human teeth is essential for consistent teaching and research in dentistry courses. Under Brazil's Transplant Law (Law No.º 9434 of 04/02/1997), which "provides for the removal of organs, tissues and parts of the human body for the purposes of transplantation and treatment", *post-mortem removal of* any part of the human body is forbidden and anyone who buys or sells tissues, organs or parts of the human body faces a penalty of 3 to 8 years in prison and a fine. The Penal Code also provides for a penalty of 1 to 3 years in prison for those who violate a grave (Article 210). **According to the National Health Council, CNS Resolution No.º 466 of 2012, which regulates the standards for the use of human beings in research, the subjects' free and informed consent is required as a form of "respect for human dignity" (BRASIL, 2016).**

Since the tooth is an organ of the human body, its origin must be known. In this context, the legal source of teeth is a Biobank of Human Teeth (BDH). In order for teeth to be used for academic purposes, they need to be granted to an institution that has a HDB. This grant must be formal and a Free and Informed Consent form must be filled out by the consenting party. This document legalizes and shows that the consenting party authorizes the granting of the material for research (NASSIF et al., 2003).

Only individuals wearing personal protective equipment may handle teeth in order to avoid cross-contamination. The preparation, selection and methods of disinfecting/sterilizing teeth can vary according to the research and, above all, the purpose for which the teeth are intended (NASSIF et al., 2003).

3.3 FUNCTIONALITY

Because it is linked to a dental university, a BDH or Biobank has various functions, including educational, scientific, clinical, social and ethical.

Considering the importance of natural teeth for undergraduate dental teaching, the Human Tooth Bank's pedagogical purpose is to make dental elements available for anatomical study, which, for example, provides a more suitable standard of sculpture for restorations, and also to meet the requirements of pre-clinical laboratory training in subjects such as Endodontics, Dentistry and Prosthodontics.

As far as scientific research is concerned, the Human Teeth Biobank would facilitate approval by the Research Ethics Committees, which have not approved research using human teeth whose origin has not been proven or legalized. This is the main objective for dental schools to set up a structured and regulated biobank, thus making material available for any and all research carried out in the academic sphere.

According to Ulson and Imparato (2008), "restorations in deciduous teeth with major coronal destruction due to fractures or caries have been a major challenge in pediatric dentistry, especially in very young patients."

According to Aguiar et al. (2000), "[...] hardness, enamel surface smoothness, translucency and the emotional factor are related to tooth loss that can be recovered by bonding dental fragments from the fractured tooth or obtained through BDH."

In the study by Avelar et al. (2009), in which they used a permanent upper central incisor and a 13-year-old male patient, they point out that, "homogenous bonding of dental fragments is an alternative to conventional restorative treatment, but this procedure requires the existence of a BHD, which offers teeth for teaching, research or clinical use, as in this case."

According to Costa et al. (2007),

The use of dental elements is extremely important for the teaching-learning process in dentistry courses. The dental element can be used in laboratory training, in research as an alternative restorative material for restorations with bonding of dental fragments in order to recompose a tooth destroyed by caries, replacing the use of materials such as amalgam, resin or porcelain, achieving better aesthetics and better color stability.

On the social side, raising public awareness of the value of the tooth as an organ; informing people of the importance of using it in scientific research and treatment. Institutions such as the BDH also perform an ethical function, as their aim is to eliminate the illegal and indiscriminate trade in human teeth. Conceptually, the tooth is an organ of the human body, so a Biobank of Human Teeth (BDH) falls under the Brazilian Transplant Law, the Brazilian Penal Code and the National Health Council.

According to ANVISA (2006), the social role of human teeth banks is to pass on information to the public and promote awareness campaigns to encourage the donation of organs, thereby creating mechanisms to curb the illegal trade in organs.

As any human cell can theoretically be cloned, the dental organ also offers cells for this purpose, such as the cells of the dental pulp and periodontal tissue. In the Dentistry course, 8% of final year students do not consider the tooth to be an organ, unaware of the fact that when a dental treatment is carried out, such as a biopulpectomy, extraction or even periodontal surgery, cells could be collected for cloning (GARBIN,et al.,2008).

3.4 RAISING TEETH FOR THE BDH

The BDH's objectives and activities must be made known to the community through programs, projects, lectures and publications in the written and/or broadcast media. Publicizing the importance of tooth grants in the form of campaigns is essential for maintaining the BDH's activities (BARRETO et al., 2003 apud Moreira et al., 2009). For Nassif et al. (2003), publicizing the importance of teeth can help increase the number of grants and, consequently, the number of activities carried out with teeth, such as research and pre-clinical laboratory studies, and reduce the trade in teeth.

Knowing how much dentists, dental students and the general population know about Biobanks, DBHs and the donation of dental organs, strategies should be devised to raise awareness about the importance of the Bank and why private collections of teeth should not be kept. Ways can also be found to encourage the donation of extracted teeth to the Biobank, contributing to its strengthening, ethical training and research (PINTO et al., 2009).

The BDH-D/UFSM's sources for collecting deciduous teeth are the teaching institution's own clinics, undergraduates, professors and researchers, the general population and local schools, where project members give talks and encourage donations (MARIN et al., 2005). The Dentistry course at ULBRA - Campus Torres, which has run a BDH since 2009, receives tooth donations from hospitals, clinics and basic health units that carry out tooth extractions, as well as from individual donations. Hence the need to make the population aware that any tooth, permanent or deciduous, and in any condition, can be donated, as everything is reused for studies (VINHOLES; FERNANDES; RITZEL; 2009).

According to Poletto et al. (2010), the recently established Biobank of Human Teeth at the Positivo University in the state of Paraná has been receiving grants of dental elements, mostly from the Health Units of the Municipal Health Department of Curitiba located in the Districts of the city.

health centers in Cidade Industrial de Curitiba and Pinheirinho. These health units are also training grounds for the institution's dental students.

3.5 TOOTH BIOBANK IN OPERATION IN BRAZIL

At USP, it all started with the slogan that was part of the campaign to donate deciduous teeth. This was in 1996, when the first of several campaigns to donate milk teeth took place on the university's website, with the aim of helping children who had lost their teeth for reasons such as caries and trauma. The campaign succeeded in becoming a tooth donation program, of which 10% were collected for the purpose of correcting the arches by gluing fragments and the remaining 90% for research (CARVALHO, 2001).

In 2003, through an extension project, a human tooth bank was set up at UNIVILLE (Universidade da Regiao de Joinville) in order to legalize the use of dental elements in research and scientific initiation projects, as well as making it easier for students and teachers to obtain teeth. In that first year, there was concern about setting up the bank, i.e. setting up the physical structure, standardizing procedural routines and starting to collect regularized dental elements for the bank's stock (ZUCOO et al., 2006).

Tooth banks or biobanks are not yet part of the routine of many dental schools in Brazil. At two meetings held at the same time as the Annual Meeting of the Brazilian Society of Dental Research in 2006 and 2007, which were attended by representatives of various dental schools in the country, the problems that many institutions face when structuring their tooth banks and/or biobanks were raised: lack of sensitivity on the part of the academic community to the subject, lack of information from the bodies that should regulate DBHs (municipal and state health surveillance secretariats, ANVISA, CROs and CFO), lack of information from the general population, which hinders grants and weakens the banks that have already been organized (PINTO et al., 2009).

CHAPTER 4

4. MATERIAL AND METHOD

4.1 MATERIAL

The materials required for the proper functioning of the Human Teeth Biobank are specified below:

The BDH at UNOESC, according to the attached project, has the following divisions: reception room (administrative), the next room is used for storage and research, in the next space, there is a sink and exhaust hood for cleaning, an autoclave for sterilization, a bacteriological culture oven and a refrigerator. A laboratory was built in accordance with current health surveillance standards. For the administration of the BDH, it is advisable to have an adjoining room with a microcomputer, filing cabinet, fax, telephone, tables, cupboards and other necessary office materials, which cost UNOESC R$5,000.00 (five thousand reais) to set up.

4.1.1 Permanent materials (laboratory equipment)

4.1.1.1 For cleaning handles

Sinks for washing material.

Spatulas, scalpel blades and scraping spatulas.

Culture oven - used in research to check that teeth are stored sterile, acquired for 3,700.00 reais through a FAPE research project entitled "Comparative study of mouthwash made with glycol extract of Punica granatum and chlorhexidine mouthwash".

Exhaustion hood - used during the cleaning and scraping of dental elements, thus avoiding the dispersal of residues from this procedure into the environment. The chapel, worth 7,900.00 (seven thousand nine hundred reais), was purchased through a FAPE research project entitled "Comparative study of mouthwash made with glycol extract of Punica granatum and chlorhexidine mouthwash".

Material sealer. 300.00 (three hundred reais).

4.1.1.2 For tooth sterilization

An autoclave without a drying process is the best way of sterilizing teeth (widely supported by scientific research), and does not significantly alter the physico-chemical properties of the tooth. It was purchased for R$2,145.44 (two thousand one hundred and forty-five reais and forty-four cents), so that it could be handled safely by undergraduates, postgraduates and researchers, after proper autoclaving and storage.

4.1.1.3 For storing teeth

Refrigerators for storing teeth, which must be kept under constant refrigeration (NASSIF, 2003), at a cost of R$1,133.10 (one thousand reais, one hundred and thirty-three cents).

Vaccine glassware, two sizes of pliers, worth R$2,500.00.

The bench for sorting and cleaning the teeth, sinks and cupboards will not generate any costs for the tooth bank project, as they come from the UNOESC university itself.

Personal biosafety materials (PPE), disinfectant solutions, ultrasound, instruments and laboratory glassware, among other materials, generated a cost of R$ 1,500.00 (one thousand five hundred reais).

4.1.2 Human resources

According to the Regulations of the BDH of UNOESC, which can be found in Annex 1 Art. 3° - The following are established as members of the Tooth Biobank:

- A general coordinator - technical coordinator Professor Léa Maria Franceschi Dallanora;
- An assistant coordinator - Professor Bruna Eliza Dedea;
- A tooth collection coordinator - Professor Acir José Dirschnabel;

- A coordinator responsible for microbiological control - Professor Fábio José Dallanora;
- An academic coordinator, representing the course, whose specific duties are set out in the regulations attached at[0] 8.

4.2 METHOD

The teeth granted to the Biobank will be used for research and will be handled in accordance with the items described below:

4.2.1 Teeth for research

The teeth granted will be treated according to the operational procedures described in the annexes, and will be used for research. They will be requested by the researchers according to their needs and after being used for the work or part of it, they must be returned to the BDH, to be reused or disposed of, according to the procedures described. In order to remove the teeth, the researchers must sign a registration form committing themselves to returning them at the end of the research. The number and group of teeth given over to each research project is established by agreement between the Human Teeth Biobank and the person responsible for the research project.

Researchers interested in acquiring teeth should therefore go to the Tooth Biobank to check that they are available. In order to use teeth from the BDH, the researcher must register, so that they can later withdraw teeth for their research. The Biobanco de Dentes provides the researcher with a form to present to the Ethics Committee and, after approval by the CEP and presentation to the Biobanco de Dentes Humanos, the teeth are released to the researcher.

4.2.2 Maintaining tooth stock

The teeth acquired by the Biobanco de Dentes Humanos (Biobank of Human Teeth) come from grants made by mail or in person and sent to the BDH, including the parents' informed consent form (TCLE) and the consent form (TA) signed by the minor. These come from agreements established with diagnostic and surgical departments, integrated clinic curricular components, pediatric dentistry curricular components, surgical extension courses and postgraduate courses in the areas of dental sciences and municipal, state and federal public services, as well as private service sectors in the region of the Association of Municipalities of the Midwest of Santa Catarina and the Association of Municipalities of the Plateau of Santa Catarina. It should be noted that the teeth will only be received if the consenting entity or patient presents and signs the ICF and the Grant Agreement, and that the teeth granted must be packed in hermetically sealed containers containing ordinary water.

CHAPTER 5

5. RESULTS AND DISCUSSION

The Tooth Biobank is a promising investment for the dental health area, which can bring benefits to the population, but it is essential to collaborate in the safe handling for learning, research and technological innovations that make use of human teeth (MORREIRA et al., 2009).

The creation of biobanks or tooth banks in Brazilian dental schools should be the best way to comply with current legislation on research involving human beings (BRASIL, 1996).

According to Pinto et al. (2009), since the 1990s it has been considered a crime to obtain organs without provenance, and the CEP does not accept research involving organs without proven origin. As a result, it has become necessary to have a place where these organs can be accessed legally, preserving the ethics and legality of the collection of these elements (CARVALHO, 2001). This is one of the factors that contributed to the establishment of the UNOESC DBH, which is characterized by a significant demand for research using human teeth and is promoted by teachers and academics.

It was also observed that the main sources of demand for teeth were dental consultations, health centers and hospitals (ZUCCO et al., 2006). The UNOESC Tooth Biobank was founded in 2011 as a tooth bank, with 10,000 teeth from the large private collections of professors and researchers and the UNOESC anatomy department, as well as grants from academics and dental surgeons. The teeth in the BDH have an informed consent form and a grant form for each batch of grants deposited in it. Currently, UNOESC's tooth biobank has a collection of 14,000 teeth, all of which have been given informed consent and are now from private clinics, dental surgeons, health centers and UNOESC's dental clinics.

The creation of the BDH required several stages, starting with the project to be drawn up for approval, then the statute or regulation according to the institution to which the Tooth Bank is linked, which must always follow ANVISA standards (IMPARATO, 2003). At UNOESC, the implementation process also went through several stages, starting with the creation of a project, which, once approved, enabled the physical space to be fitted out in accordance with the instructions described in the book Banco de Dentes Humanos (Human Tooth Bank) by José Carlos Imparato e Cois, and the ANVISA instructions. Secondly, the tooth grants were catalogued, and finally, the legal part was studied, in which the regulations of the UNOESC HDB were created, following the laws and statutes of the institution, currently, the UNOESC HDB is seeking its regulation with CONEP.

A functioning DBH must have regulations or statutes, which specify all the documents necessary for its full operation (NASSIF et al., 2003). These regulations state who is responsible for the DBH. In the case of the DBH at UNOESC, we have regulations as shown in Annex 1, because UNOESC believes that the tooth biobank is an extension of the dentistry course and is governed by it, rather than a separate body with a statute. According to Article 3 of the regulations, the BDH has a general coordinator, an assistant coordinator who is a lecturer on the course and is responsible for the Tooth Biobank, two assistant technical lecturers, one responsible for microbiological control and one for the collection process, and an academic coordinator (a student on the dentistry course) who also works with two trainees who are responsible for receiving, cleaning and storing the teeth in the bank, under the supervision of the general coordinator.

According to Article 9 of the regulations, the UNOESC Tooth Biobank has its own book, with numbered pages and opening and closing dates initialed by the competent health authority, which is used to register consenting patients and their registered identity card, and another book with the same characteristics for registering patients who have been granted teeth, or requesting professors.

According to Ferreira et al. (2003), the tooth belonging to the BDH must have a proven origin, by means of a grant agreement. The BDH must be organized and have careful functionality so that everything can be carried out within the rules established by the institution's regulations, not forgetting the Free and Informed Consent document for the use of the teeth and signed by the same. At UNOESC's BDH, teeth are received by means of a specific consent form for each location, one for the individual consenting to the tooth; one for deciduous teeth, where the parents or guardians are the consenting parties in this case along with the minor's consent form, another specific form for private DC collections, and finally, a specific form for health departments and the like.

The BDHs linked to the Dentistry Courses reduce the risk of cross-infections from incorrect handling of dental organs and organize the supply of these elements to undergraduate and postgraduate students (POLETTO et al., 2010). Therefore, the BDH at UNOESC receives the grant of the dental element, which after being catalogued goes through a scraping and cleaning session and is then packaged in an appropriate and sterilized package, and finally stored in distilled water, and will be available for dental research.

According to the study by Zucco et al. (2006), 66.6% of the students handled teeth without personal protective equipment (lab coat, cap, gloves, mask and goggles), despite the fact that 86.8% of the students interviewed knew that blood-borne pathogens transmissible to humans can exist in the root pulp and periodontal tissues.

In agreement with Costa et al. (2007), it is not enough just to know where extracted human teeth come from and how they are used in the teaching-learning process; another important issue is to know which decontamination and storage procedures are being used.

According to Zucco et al. (2006), surprisingly, during their research, they found that students are aware of what the tooth bank is and yet there was a great deal of resistance on the part of the students when it comes to donating teeth to the biobank. This may have been due to a lack of knowledge about the activities of the biobank and the rules of procedure for donating and removing dental elements. To date, the BDH at UNOESC has received around 1,186 teeth extracted in the course's clinics, around 2,890 from teachers and students, around 1980 from health departments in other municipalities, around 9,185 teeth from the curricular components of dentistry, endodontics, anatomy and around 500 teeth from the course's anatomy laboratory, and around 2,000 teeth for research by researchers in their theses, specializations, master's degrees and doctorates.

It is known that it takes time for the culture of valuing the tooth as an organ to be formed, which is why it is essential that dental schools include information on this subject in their curricula and that more scientific studies are developed (PINTO et al., 2009).

However, despite exposing the process of implementing the BDH in universities, it is also necessary for academics themselves to publicize it to society, with the aim of making people aware that granting teeth to the BDH will bring benefits to society, to academics and to the research carried out within universities.

FINAL CONSIDERATIONS

The implementation of human tooth banks and biobanks in universities fulfills an important ethical, moral and scientific function, storing teeth in accordance with biosafety standards, the necessary organization and its functionality, encouraging its importance in the research scenarios of Dentistry courses, encouraging and convincing academics that this information should reach society, thus highlighting the need and importance of regulation by CONEP for the Dentistry course at UNOESC.

REFERENCES

1- NATIONAL HEALTH SURVEILLANCE AGENCY (ANVISA). **Dental services:** risk prevention and control. Brasilia: 2006. Available at http://www.anvisa.gov.br/servicosaude/manuais /manual odonto.pdf> Accessed on: 07 Sep. 2011.

2- AGUIAR, Karen. C. F. M de, et al. **Homogenous Bonding:** Alternative Technique for Fractured Anterior Teeth. Revista Gaúcha de Odontologia, v.48, n.3, p. 153-154,jul/ago/set.2000

3- AVELAR, Felipe Morando; PENIDO, Cláudia Valéria de Sousa Resende; CRUZ, Roberval de Almeida; Sérgio PENIDO, Milton Sergio Martins de Oliveira. Homogenous bonding of a tooth fragment in a permanent maxillary central incisor - clinical case report. RFO, v. 14, n. 1, p. 66- 70, January/April 2009

4- BEGOSSO, M. P.; IMPARATO, J. C. P.; DUARTE, D. A. Current status of the organization of human tooth banks in dental schools in Brazil. *RPG Rev. Pós Grad.*, v. 8,n. 1. 23-28, Jan./Mar. 2001.

5- BRAZIL. Ordinance No.^{0} 904/00, Ministry of Health, August 16, 2000. 2000. **Official Journal of the Union**. Available at: <www.conselho.saude.gov.br>. Accessed on: May 3, 2016.

6- BRAZIL. Resolution no. 196, of October 16, 1996. **Diário Oficial da Uniäo**, Brasilia, DF, October 16, 1996. Available at: <www.conselho.saude.gov.br>. Accessed on: 03 May 2016.

7- BRAZIL. Resolution no. 441, of May 12, 2011. **Official Gazette da Uniäo**, Brasilia, DF, May 12, 2011. Available at: <www.conselho.saude.gov.br>. Accessed on: 05 May 2016.

8- CARVALHO, Cíntia. **Teeth in the Crosshairs of Ethics.** Revista Brasileira de Odontologia, v. 58, n. 2, p. 108-111, mar/abr.2001.

9- COSTA, S. M.; et al. Human teeth in dental education: origin, use, decontamination and storage by UNIMONTES academics. **ABENO Journal.** Brasilia. v.7, n.1, p.6-12. 2007.

10- FERREIRA, E. L. et al. **Tooth Bank**: Ethics and Legality in Dental Teaching, Research and Treatment. Rev. Bras. Odontol., Rio de Janeiro, v. 60, n. 2, p. 120-122, mar/abr. 2003.

11- GARBIN, C. A. S. **Dental students' perceptions of cloning, organ donation and tooth banking.** Revista Pós Graduado, v.15, n. 4, p. 255-60.2008.

12- IMPARATTO, J. C. P. - Banco de Dentes Humanos - Editora Maio. Curitiba. 2003.

13- MAGGIONI. A.R.; et al. Human tooth bank in the perception of academics at the Faculty of Dentistry of the Fluminense Federal University. **Revista Fluminense de Odontologia**. v.4, n.33. p.27-30. 2010.

14- MELO, C.R.O. **Human tooth bank in a teaching institution:** importance, implementation and operation. Brazilian Dental Association. Federal University of Minas Gerais. Belo Horizonte, 2005. 35 p.

15- MOREIRA, L et al. **Human Tooth Bank for Teaching and Research in Dentistry.** Rev. Fac. Odontol. Porto Alegre, v. 50, n. 1, p. 34-37, jan./abr., 2009.

16- NASSIF, A. C. S. et al. **Structure of a Human Tooth Bank.** Pesq. Odontol. Bras., Sáo Paulo, v. 17, p.70-74, May 2003. PEREIRA, Daylis Quinto. Human tooth banks in Brazil: a literature review. **Revista da Abeno,** Londrina, v. 12, n. 2, p.178-184,

2012.

17-   PEREIRA, D. Q. **Survey of tooth banks in dentistry courses in Brazil and experience with the creation of a human tooth bank at the State University of Feira de Santana.**
Bahia. 2012. 110 f. Thesis (Doctorate) - Medicine Course, Bahia Medical School, Salvador, 2012.

18-   PINTO, L. S. et al. **Popular, Academic and Professional Knowledge about the Human Tooth Bank.** Pesq Bras Odontoped Clin Integr, Joáo Pessoa, 9(1):101-106,jan./abr. 2009.

19-   POLETTO, M. M. et al. **Human Tooth Bank: Socio-Cultural Profile of a Donor Group.** RGO, Porto Alegre, v. 58, n.1, p. 91-94, jan./mar. 2010.

20-   ULSON, Raquel Cristina Barbosa, IMPARATO, José Carlos Pettorossi. **Mouth Rehabilitation by Fragment Bonding in Deciduous Teeth** Publ. UEPG Ci. Biol. Saúde, Ponta Grossa, v.14,n.l, p. 23-28, mar. 2008.

21-   VANZELLI, M.; RAMOS, D. L. de P.; IMPARATO, J. C. P. Appreciation of the tooth as an organ. In: IMPARATO, José Carlos Pettorossi. **Human tooth bank.** Curitiba: Editora Maio, 2003. p. 33-37.

22-   ZANATTA, C. et al. Implanted from the human teeth bank (BDH) of the dentistry course at the University of Western Santa Catarina. **Unoesc & Ciencia [online]**, Joa^aba, v. 5, n.1, jul. 2014.

23-   ZUCCO, D.; KOBE, R.; FABRE, C.; MADEIRA, L.; BARATTO FILHO, F.. **Evaluation of the Level of Knowledge of UNIVILLE Dentistry Course Students on the Utilization of Extracted Teeth in the Undergraduate Program and the Tooth Bank.** Revista Sul-Brasileira de Odontologia v.3,n.1, 2006 - 55.

ANNEXES

1. **LEGAL OPINION № 082/2010/PJG.**
2. **LETTER FROM THE RECTOR.**
3. **TERMS:**
   3.1 TERM OF INSTITUTIONAL RESPONSIBILITY (TRI): INSTITUTIONAL DECLARATION OF TECHNICAL AND FINANCIAL RESPONSIBILITY FOR SETTING UP AND MAINTAINING THE BIOBANK, PART OF THE DEVELOPMENT PROTOCOL;
   3.2 INFORMED CONSENT FORM;
   3.3 INFORMED CONSENT FORM FOR MINORS;
   3.4 CONSENT FORM;
   3.5 TERM OF CONCESSION FOR HUMAN TEETH - INDIVIDUAL;
   3.6 TERM OF CONCESSION FOR HUMAN TEETH - FROM THE DENTAL SURGEON;
   3.7 TERM OF COMMITMENT TO SERVE;
   3.8 TERM OF RETURN OF HUMAN TEETH AFTER THE END OF THE RESEARCH;
   a. MODEL FOR REQUESTING TEETH FROM COORDINATION;
   b. TEMPLATE FOR A CONTROL SHEET FOR ASSIGNED TEETH;
   c. DECLARATION TO THE RESEARCH ETHICS COMMITTEE.
4. **OPERATING PROCEDURES.... _______..**
5. **BOOK OF CONCESSION RECORDS.**
6. **MINUTES.**

2.REGULATIONS OF THE HUMAN TEETH BIOBANK OF THE DENTISTRY COURSE UNIVERSIDADE DO OESTE DE SANTA CATARINA (UNOESC)

Art. I° The Biobank of Human Teeth of the Dentistry Course of the Universidade do Oeste de Santa Catarina - Unoesc, Joa^aba Campus, is a sector located on the premises of the Dentistry Course of the Universidade do Oeste de Santa Catarina, responsible for collecting, preparing, disinfecting, handling, seating, preserving, storing, loaning and administering the teeth provided by the general population, as well as being responsible for its own dissemination.

Sole paragraph - This sector will only operate with the mandatory presence of the dental surgeon in charge (general coordinator and/or assistant), or of the technical coordinators who are legally qualified and have signed a term of responsibility with the competent health authority.

Art. 2 The objectives of the Human Teeth Biobank are:

I - Research Objective: to lend and/or transfer available teeth to undergraduates, postgraduates and researchers in general to enable scientific research to be carried out, such as transplants, aesthetic veneers, fixed adhesive prostheses, fragment bonding and others.

II - General objective: to value the tooth as an organ and to raise awareness among the lay community, academics and dental surgeons of the cultural, bioethical, social, legal and moral importance of the existence of a Human Tooth Biobank, as an organ bank, preserving the teeth granted with the appropriate means, supported by scientific research.

§ 10 - The Biobanco de Dentes Humanos or its members, collaborators and academics are forbidden from receiving or paying any money or advantages, under any title whatsoever, for withdrawing or delivering the organs granted.

§ 20 - Members of the Human Teeth Biobank are prohibited from directly providing dental care to patients at its headquarters.

§ 30 - Authorization to operate the Unoesc Human Teeth Biobank will be requested from the competent health authority by the dental surgeon and/or professor in charge, in an application that must be accompanied by the Human Teeth Biobank regulations.

§40 - The granting of teeth will be defined by those responsible for the Human Teeth Biobank, after analysis of the Research Project.

Art. 30 - The following are established as members of the Human Teeth Biobank: I- a general coordinator; II- an auxiliary coordinator; III- two technical coordinators, represented by four professors from the Dentistry Course and; IV- an academic coordinator, represented by an academic from the Dentistry Course.

§io. The Human Teeth Biobank must maintain a duly qualified and legally qualified technical staff, in sufficient numbers for the perfect execution of its activities.

§20. In the event of a change of personnel or tenure of professors working in the Biobanco, the change will be immediately communicated to the CEP/CONEP System, in accordance with CNS Resolution 441 of 2011, item 3.IV.

Art. 4º - The functions of the general coordinator are:

I   - to represent the Human Teeth Biobank;

II   - chairing meetings;

III   - to comply with and enforce these Regulations and the Internal Regulations of Unoesc;

IV   - sign documents, letters and newsletters relating to the sector;

V   - take care of this sector that serves philanthropic activity;

VI   - appoint representatives;

VII   - represent the Biobank of Human Teeth in solemnities and public acts;

VIII   - vote in meetings;

IX   - to keep the entity in good standing with the competent health authority;

X   - controlling the processes of collecting, preparing, disinfecting, handling, selecting, preserving, storing, granting and administering the teeth granted.

Art. 50 - The assistant coordinator's duties are:

I   - to represent the Human Teeth Biobank;

II   - chairing meeting sessions in the absence of the general coordinator;

III   - comply with and enforce these regulations and the Internal Regulations of Unoesc;

IV   - sign documents, letters and newsletters relating to the sector in the absence of the general coordinator;

V   - represent the Biobank of Human Teeth in solemnities and public acts;

VI   - vote in meetings.

Art. 6º - The technical coordinators have the following responsibilities:

f - sign the book of concessions, reception and technical-dental file;

II   - to keep the entity in good standing with the competent health authority;

III   - controlling the processes of collection, preparation, disinfection, handling, selection, preservation, storage, cessation and administration of the teeth granted;

IV   - to replace the general coordinator in his or her functions, as long as this is regulated by the competent health authority;

V   - vote in meetings.

Art. 70 - The academic coordinator has the following duties:

I   - to establish relations between the Human Teeth Biobank and the student body;

II   - sign documents, letters and newsletters relating to the sector;

III   - vote in meetings;

Art. 80 - The Human Tooth Biobank is equipped with: a suitable portable and sterilized thermal unit with the necessary instruments for handling the tooth provided by the legally qualified dental surgeon(s), a refrigerator, aprons, caps, gloves, masks, goggles and containers with sterilizing solution, numbered and properly identified, in accordance with what is established by the competent health authority.

§ lo - The Human Teeth Biobank must have adequate infrastructure in terms of water, sewage and electricity services, at the discretion of the competent health authority, which must be kept in perfect order and hygiene.

§ 2º - The working establishment must have a floor made of smooth, resistant and impermeable material, light-colored walls and partitions with a bar at least two meters high, made of smooth and impermeable material, as established by the competent health authority.

§ Paragraph 30 - The establishment must have rooms or compartments separated up to the ceiling by uninterrupted walls or partitions, with a minimum area of ten square meters each, intended for an administrative unit with reception and archive and a laboratory.

§ 40- The laboratory must have light-colored floors and walls, covered with smooth, impermeable material that is resistant to the products used for asepsis.

§ 50 - The workplace must have an independent entrance, not serve as a passage to another location, and its premises may not be used for other purposes.

Art. 90 Art. 90 - The Human Teeth Biobank must have: I- a book with numbered pages, with opening and closing terms duly initialed by the competent health authority, for the registration of consenting patients and the number of their Identity Card; II- a book with numbered pages, with opening and closing terms initialed by the competent health authority, for the registration of teeth granted or of requesting professors.

Sole Paragraph - The books referred to in the *heading of* this article must be strictly up to date and must remain on the premises of the company.

Human Teeth Biobank and will be shown to the competent health authority whenever requested.

Art. 10-0 Biobanco de Dentes Humanos will send the competent health authority a list of the previous year's consenters by the end of March, together with the names of those responsible *for* the teeth granted for scientific research, as well as documentation regarding the approval of the research carried out, in the form of authorization from the Research Support Sector and approval from the institution's Research Ethics Committee.

Art. 11 - The teeth stored in the Human Teeth Biobank come from grants made by correspondence or in person, upon presentation and signature of the informed consent form, in accordance with the annexes to these Regulations, with prior performance, at the time of the grant, of all the screening tests for diagnosis of infection and infestation required by regulatory standards issued by the Ministry of Health.

§ 1º - Teeth sent for concession, until they reach the Human Teeth Biobank, must be packed in a hermetically sealed container with ordinary water.

§ Paragraph 2 The concession may be revoked by the consenting party or those legally responsible at any time prior to its implementation.

Art. 12-0 The Human Teeth Biobank will indiscriminately respond to requests for teeth made by legally qualified and duly qualified dental surgeons or researchers, following the chronological order of registration in the appropriate book, provided that the purpose of the request is approved by the members of the committee responsible for the Human Teeth Biobank.

Sole paragraph. In the event of a duly proven emergency, the order of registration may be disregarded.

§ Iº -Empréslimo is carried out when a researcher needs more denles and doesn't read them, he makes a request to the Human Denles Biobank of the University of Oesle de Sanla Catarina filling in all the questions required by the coordinators of the Human Denles Biobank.

§ 20- After approval by the CEPs of the institutions involved and with all the paperwork completed in accordance with the requirements of the BDH, the samples will be sent to the researcher together with the Biological Material Transfer Agreement (duly completed).

Art. 13 - In the event of the closure of the Human Dengue Biobank's facilities, the competent health authority must be notified and, in compliance with the procedural rules, its assets will be transferred to other human blood biobanks and the consenting party will be informed of the loss or destruction of their biological samples, the closure of the biobank and the transfer of biological material between biobanks, where appropriate.

Article 14 - The license to operate the Human Dengue Biobank will be renewed annually in accordance with the legislation in force in the city where the entity is based and in accordance with the rules of the Health Surveillance Agency.

Sole paragraph. The technical coordinator must present his or her work agreement with the facility where the Human Dengue Biobank is located, so that it can be registered with the health agency.

Art. 15-0 These regulations may be amended in whole or in part if so requested by half plus one of the members with voting rights.

Art. 16-0 These regulations shall enter into force on the date of their approval.

Joa^aba,___ de de.

President of Consun

3.Good Practices Manual for the Human Teeth Biobank - BDH

1. Purpose.

The purpose of UNOESC's human teeth biobank is to correctly and sterilely store the dental elements given to this laboratory, which will be used specifically for life sciences research.

2. Captured from dental elements.

The dental elements (teeth) stored in UNOESC's biobank come from grants, collected from private clinics, health centers and the institution's dental clinics. Teeth are also collected by students in their communities through grants from patients.

The consent forms are stored in the Biobank's archives and only the general and auxiliary coordinators and the academic coordinator have access to this data, which is secured through differentiated access passwords that are changed monthly, in order to avoid the process of coding and decoding and the identification of the research subject by unauthorized personnel.

The teeth (biological material) are stored in locked cabinets in a specific room, with access restricted to personnel authorized to handle the teeth.

The entire building where the Biobank is located is monitored by cameras and has 24-hour security guards (outsourced service). Thus, the secrecy and confidentiality of the consenters' data and access to the stored samples and the information associated with these samples is in accordance with MS Ordinance No.^{0} 2.201 of 2011, Section III, Article 23, § 2º

3. Destination of stored dental elements

3.1 Biobank Research Activities.

The teeth are handed over upon request in the appropriate form for the activities carried out in research at the institution or outside it, in accordance with the terms of mutual cooperation, and will only be forwarded after the TTBM (Term of Transfer of Biological Material) has been signed.

4. Located in the Human Teeth Biobank.

The human teeth biobank is located in the Dentistry course, Campus II in the city of Joa^aba (SC) in its own room, on the first floor, with conditions for receiving, cleaning, preparing, storing and dispensing dental elements.

5. Documents inherent to the UNOESC Biobank.

5.1 Documentary terms.

5.1.1 APPENDIX I - Terms and conditions for the use of human teeth (ICF, ICF for minors and Term of Assent (TA)).

5.1.2 ANNEX II - Declaration of disposal of human teeth.

5.1.3 ANNEX III - Model for requesting human teeth for research

5.1.4 ANNEX IV - Term of communication regarding the sterilization process of Dental Elements.

5.1.5 ANNEX V - Term of commitment to quote.

5.1.6 ANNEX VI - Declaration to the Research Ethics Committee 1 and 2

5.1.7 ANNEX VII - Terms of grant (student, CD)

5.1.8 ANNEX VIII - Internal control sheet.

5.1.9 ANNEX IX - Term of Institutional Responsibility **(TRI)**

5.1.10 ANNEX X - Management Responsibility Statement

5.1.11 ANNEX XI - Biological Material Transfer Agreement (BTMT)

5.1.12 ANNEX XII - Letter of Notice to the Consenting Party for the Subsequent Disposal of Biological Material.

5.2 Standard Operating Procedures.

5.2.1 How to draw up the BDH's Standard Operating Procedures.

5.2.2 POP of capture.

5.2.3 Transportation SOP (receiving and shipping).

5.2.4 SOP for cleaning, preparation and selection of incoming dental elements.

5.2.5 SOP for packaging, sterilization and storage.

5.2.6 Loan and disposal SOP.

>   This procedure includes the tooth removal form and the return form with a numbered record in the appropriate book.

5.2.7 SOP for microbiological quality control.

>   This procedure includes the microbiological methodology, frequency and form of statistical analysis to guarantee sterile quality.

5.2.8 SOP for selecting trainees.

<u>ANNEX I</u>

INFORMED CONSENT FORM

You are being invited as a volunteer to donate your tooth to the biobank of the Universidade do Oeste de Santa Catarina.

The reason for proposing to grant this tooth is that it is one of the most important elements in research into restorative techniques, restorative materials and more. Research is justified in order to improve the quality of work in the dental field. The aim of this project is to collect teeth to provide the means for research within the dentistry course at UNOESC.

Data collection procedures will take place as follows: A control will be carried out through the terms of concession, with the data of the consenter, a container will be provided for the collection of the tooth (biological material), following all the rules of biosafety. The tooth will be sent to the biobank and will be catalogued according to the consenter's record. Whenever the consenter wants to access their data, they will be allowed to do so. And if they want to remove their tooth from the biobank, it will be given to them.

Your participation in this project will not generate any kind of discomfort, the risk of your participation will be minimal, but the benefit that will be obtained, for example by testing new restorative materials, will be of enormous value within dentistry.

FORM OF MONITORING AND ASSISTANCE:

Your grant, in this case the tooth, will be deposited in the Biobank for an indefinite period of time, and any costs generated by this deposit will be borne by the institution or the researcher. Your tooth may be used in various research projects using restorative techniques and materials, and with each new research project that is started on your tooth or that uses data stored where your tooth has been used, you will be notified immediately and will have complete freedom to consent to or stop the research. When a tooth is transferred between biobanks due to the end of the biobank's existence or shared research, or when your biological material is lost, discarded or destroyed, you will be notified and you will be free to consent to or stop the process by withdrawing your tooth.

Please tick your consent option below:

( )- A new consent form is required for each study, ( )- A new consent form is not required for each study, in accordance with CNS Resolution no.^{0} 441 of 2011.

GUARANTEE OF CLARIFICATION, FREEDOM OF REFUSAL AND GUARANTEE OF CONFIDENTIALITY:

You can ask for clarification about the research and where your tooth is at any stage of the study. You are free to refuse to participate, withdraw your consent or stop participating in the research at any time, for reasons of embarrassment or otherwise. Your participation is voluntary and refusal to participate will not result in any penalty or loss of benefits. The researcher(s) will treat your identity with professional standards of confidentiality. The results of the studies on your tooth will be sent to you and will remain confidential. Your name or material indicating your participation will not be released without your permission. You will not be identified in any publication that may result from this study. This form is printed and signed in two copies, one copy will be given to you and the other will be kept in the UNOESC biobank.

COSTS OF PARTICIPATION, COMPENSATION AND INDEMNIFICATION:

Participation in this project will not cost you anything and no financial compensation will be provided. If you suffer any damage as a result of this research, you should contact the general coordinator of the biobank.

STATEMENT BY THE PARTICIPATING SUBJECT OR THE PERSON RESPONSIBLE FOR THE PARTICIPATING SUBJECT:

For vulnerable individuals such as children, adolescents, prisoners, Indians, people with mental capacity or reduced autonomy, they must have a legal representative, without prejudice to their authorization.

I, ...,(name of legal representative, if

Impressão dactiloscópica

I have been informed of the objectives of the above grant in a clear and detailed manner and have clarified my doubts. I know that at any time I may request further information and/or withdraw my consent. Those responsible for the Biobanks above have assured me that all my data will be kept confidential. If I have any questions, I can call the general coordinator of the biobank, a professor who is the general coordinator of the BDH, resident, with the CPF and telephone number, email, or the assistant coordinator, a professor who is resident, with the CPF, telephone number, email, or contact the Ethics Committee for Research on Human Beings at Unoesc/Hust, Rua Getúlio Vargas, n^0 2125, Bairro Flor da Serra, 89600000- Joa^aba - SC, Phone: 49-3551-2012. I declare that I agree to give up my tooth. I have received a copy of this informed consent form and have been given the opportunity to read it and clarify my doubts.

Signature of the consenting subject or **fingerprint.**

Signature:
Legible name:
Address:
Email:
RG.
Phone:
Date /
Signature of the researcher responsible
Date//
IMPORTANT: PRINT THE FORM IN TWO TIMES, one
copy to be kept by the consenting subject and the other by the
researcher responsible. The research subject or his/her representative, if applicable, must initial all the pages of the Informed Consent Form and sign the last page. The researcher in charge must do the same, initial all the sheets of the ICF and sign the last page of the form.

Minor Participant

INFORMED CONSENT FORM

The minor, under your responsibility, is being asked to volunteer to donate a tooth to the biobank of the University of Western Santa Catarina. The aim of the biobank is to provide teeth for research in the life sciences.

The reason for proposing to grant this tooth is that it is an important element in research into restorative techniques, restorative materials and more. Research is justified in order to improve the quality of work in the dental field. The aim of this project is to collect teeth to provide the means for research within the dentistry course at UNOESC.

Data collection procedures will take place as follows: A control will be carried out through the terms of concession, with the consenter's data, a container will be provided for the collection of the tooth (biological material), following all biosafety rules. The tooth will be sent to the biobank and will be catalogued according to the consenter's record. Whenever the consenter wants to access their data, they will be allowed to do so. And if they want to remove their tooth from the biobank, it will be given to them.

To take part in this grant, the minor under your responsibility will not be charged anything or receive any financial advantage. They will be informed in any way they wish and will be free to participate or refuse to participate. You, as the minor's guardian, can withdraw your consent or stop the minor's participation at any time. The child's participation is voluntary and refusal to participate will not result in any penalty or change in the way the child is treated by the researcher, who will treat the child's identity with professional standards of confidentiality. The child will not be identified in any way. Participation in this project will not generate any discomfort, this grant presents minimal risk, that is, the same risk that exists in routine activities such as talking, bathing, reading, etc., but the benefit that will be obtained, for example by testing new restorative materials, will be of enormous value within dentistry. Even so, the minor has the right to compensation in the event of any damage caused by the research.

FORM OF MONITORING AND ASSISTANCE:

Your grant, in this case the tooth, will be deposited in the Biobank for an indefinite period of time, and any costs generated by this deposit will be borne by the institution or the researcher. Your tooth may be used in various research projects using restorative techniques and materials, and with each new research project that is started on your tooth or that uses data stored where your tooth has been used, you will be notified immediately and will have complete freedom to consent to or stop the research. When your tooth is transferred between biobanks due to the end of the biobank's existence or shared research, or when your biological material is lost, discarded or destroyed, you will be notified and you will be free to consent to or stop the process by withdrawing your tooth.

Please check your consent option below: ( )- A new consent form is required for each study, ( )- A new consent form is not required for each study, according to CNS Resolution[0] 441 of 2011.

GUARANTEE OF CLARIFICATION, FREEDOM OF REFUSAL AND GUARANTEE OF CONFIDENTIALITY:

You can ask for clarification about the research and where your tooth is at any stage of the study. You are free to refuse to participate, withdraw your consent or stop participating in the research at any time, for reasons of embarrassment or otherwise. Your participation is voluntary and refusal to participate will not result in any penalty or loss of benefits. The researcher(s) will treat your identity with professional standards of confidentiality.

The results will be made available to you at the end of any research where the tooth in our care is used. The name or material indicating the participation of the minor will not be released without their permission. The data and instruments used in the research will be stored with the researcher responsible for a period of 5 years, after which time they will be destroyed. The minor will not be identified in any publication that may result from this study. When you reach the age of 18, we will send you a consent form for the material you have given to this Biobank.

This form is printed and signed in two copies, one copy will be given to you and the other will be kept in the UNOESC biobank.

COSTS OF PARTICIPATION, COMPENSATION AND INDEMNIFICATION:

Participation in this project will not entail any costs for you or the child under your responsibility and no financial compensation will be provided. In the event of any damage arising from this research, you should contact the general coordinator of the biobank.

DECLARED BY THE PARTICIPATING SUBJECT OR THE PERSON RESPONSIBLE FOR THE PARTICIPATING SUBJECT:

For vulnerable individuals such as children, adolescents, prisoners, Indians, people with mental capacity or reduced autonomy, they must have a legal representative, without prejudice to their authorization.

I, , bearer of identity document , responsible for the minor (For vulnerable individuals such as children, adolescents, prisoners, Indians, people with mental capacity or reduced autonomy) , have been informed of the objectives of this grant in a clear and detailed manner and have clarified my doubts. I understand that at any time I can request further information from the general coordinator of the biobank, professor and resident BDH general coordinator, with CPF and telephone number.

email or with the assistant coordinator teacher , resident with

CPFtelephone _________________ email, _____________________ or with the Ethics Committee for Research with Human Beings at Unoesc/Hust, telephone: (49) 3551-2012. I am aware that I can change the decision of the minor under my responsibility to take part in the study if I so wish. I have received a copy of this informed consent form and have been given the opportunity to read it and clarify my doubts.

Signature of consenting subject or **fingerprint**. Signature:

Legible name:

Address:

Email:

RG.

Phone:

Date /   **Signature of researcher responsible**

Date /   **TERM OF ASSENT (TA) CHILD 07 ALL YEARS**

You are being invited as a volunteer to hand over your baby tooth to UNOESC's TOOTH BIOBANK.

- At the university we have an appropriate place to store your tooth until you want to.
- Your tooth will be used to study new materials to treat teeth and thus improve the health of children's mouths.

In order for the human tooth biobank to comply with Brazilian law, we will work with your tooth as follows:

- Once the teeth have been delivered, they will be washed and stored in labeled jars in the biobank.

To take part in this study, your guardian must authorize you to do so and sign a consent form:

- There will be no cost to you.
- You will not receive payment for the tooth(s).
- You will be notified about the surveys if you wish.
- You are free to participate or refuse to participate in the research.
- Your guardian can withdraw consent or stop your participation at any time.
- Your participation is voluntary.
- You can withdraw from the survey at any time.
- You will not be identified in any publication.
- The results of the survey will be available to you at the end of the survey.
- The information used in the research will be kept by the researcher responsible for a period of 5 years, after which time it will be destroyed.

Impressão dactiloscópica
Impressão dactiloscópica

This consent form is printed in two copies, one of which will be kept by the researcher responsible and the other will be given to you.

Eu\ , z x ; ------------------- .   , -------------------------------------- ...   . T-■   '

Identity card holder ____ (if you already have one)

document), I have been clearly informed that my tooth will be stored in the Unoesc tooth biobank. I understand that I can request further information from the researcher in charge, prof. Léa Maria Franceschi Dallanora, telephone: 49 991042226, or Unoesc, telephone (49) 3551-2012. I am aware that my guardian can change my decision to take part in the research if they wish. With my guardian's consent already signed, I declare that I agree to lend my tooth. I have received a copy of this consent form and have been given the opportunity to read it and clarify my doubts.

,de de 20.

Signature of the minor or fingerprint.

Legible name:

Address:

RG.

Phone:

Date//

Signature of the researcher responsible

Legible name:
Address:
Phone:
Date//

Impressão
dactiloscópica

CONSENT FORM (TA) - ADOLESCENTS
AGED 12 TO 17

You are being invited as a volunteer to donate your tooth to
the Biobank of the University of Western Santa Catarina. In this project we have an appropriate place to store your tooth for an indefinite period of time, if you so decide.

The reason why we created the biobank, and why we're applying for it now, is to have teeth available for research into dental materials and new techniques for restoring teeth, with a view to the evolution of dentistry.

To ensure that the human teeth biobank complies with the laws of Brazil, we will adopt the following procedure(s): the teeth will be stored in the biobank after they have been collected (granted), but beforehand they will be treated in accordance with the biobank's operating procedures, and afterwards they will be stored in identified jars which allow the tooth to be located after the grant.

To take part in this project, your guardian must authorize you to do so and sign a consent form. There will be no cost to you, nor will you receive any financial advantage. You will be informed in any way you wish and you are free to participate or refuse. Your guardian can withdraw consent or stop your participation at any time. Your participation is voluntary and refusal to participate will not result in any penalty or change in the way you are treated by the researcher who will treat your identity with professional standards of confidentiality. You will not be identified in any publication. This project presents minimal risk, i.e. the same risk that exists in routine activities such as talking, bathing, reading, etc. Nevertheless, you have the right to compensation in the event of any damage caused by the research.

The results will be made available to you at the end of the study. Your name or any material indicating your participation will not be released without the permission of the person responsible for you. **When you turn 18, we will send you a consent form for the material you have given to this Biobank.** The data and instruments used in the research will be stored with the researcher responsible for a period of 5 years, after which time they will be destroyed. This consent form is printed in two copies, one of which will be kept by the researcher responsible and the other will be given to you.

I, , bearer of an identity document (if I already have one), have been clearly informed of the objectives of this study. I understand that at any time I may request further information from the general coordinator of the biobank, professor, ___ general coordinator   of   the
BDH. a, bearer of CPF and telephone ,email or with the assistant coordinator teacher, resident bearer of CPFtelephone
email or with

Unoesc and Hust Human Research Ethics Committee, telephone (49) 3551-2012. I am aware that my guardian may modify the decision to participate in the research if he/she so wishes. With my guardian's consent already signed, I declare that I agree to give up my tooth. I have received a copy of this consent form and have been given the opportunity to read it and clarify my doubts. ,de de 20.

Signature of the minor or fingerprint.
Legible name:
Address:
Email:

RG.
Phone:
Date//

Signature of the researcher responsible
Legible name:
Address:
Email:
Phone:
Date//

ANNEX II
RETURN OF HUMAN TEETH

I, , bearer of ID,   am
returning teeth to the BIOBANK OF
HUMAN TEETH OF THE COURSE OF ODONTOLOGY OF THE UNIVERSITY OF THE
WEST OF SANTA CATARINA - UNOESC, which were used in the research called
", so that it can be disposed of in accordance with the current rules recommended by the
National Health Council (CNS).
Joa^aba, 20.

____

                                                                                    Signature

ANNEX III

Letterhead of your university or study center.

Example: Federal University of Rio Grande do Sul.

Dentistry course

Requested

Coordinator of the Dentistry Course at the University of the West of Santa Catarina -
UNOESC
Subject: Request for human teeth for research purposes.
Dear Prof[1] , in order to develop the project
entitled____
, in progress or approved by the Research Ethics Committee of the   Faculty of Dentistry
of ____
we hereby request the Tooth Biobank of your Institution.

In advance, we would like to point out that we will duly note the origin of the teeth
used in our research.

Thank you in advance for your attention and my best wishes. Name of applicant and
position (if held) Name of supervisor

ANNEX IV
NOTICE REGARDING THE
STERILIZATION PROCESS OF
DENTAL ELEMENTS

Dear researcher: Many studies have shown that the storage solution of teeth used *in "in vitro"*
or *"in situ"* studies can interfere with the final results, depending on the type of medium used.
As there is still no consensus in the literature regarding the best storage medium and also in
order not to interfere with the results of your research, the HUMAN TOOTH BIOBANK OF
THE COURSE OF ODONTOLOGY OF THE UNIVERSITY OF THE WEST OF SANTA
CATARINA - UNOESC has as its storage protocol for your teeth the use of distilled water

without preservative additives of any kind.

The dental elements you are receiving are STERILE by autoclaving.

Even if the material is sterile, handle the dental elements using PPE.

This term is your certificate that the dental elements contained in the bottle have been sterilized as long as they have not been tampered with by removing the aluminium seal or perforating the rubber cap.

Joa^aba,de de.

Responsible for the BDH at UNOESC

For use in the biobank

Registration of the concession term number:book page

Electronic protocol number: _______________________________

ANNEX V
CITATION UNDERTAKING

I, (name of applicant) RG ., hereby commit myself to the BDH/UNOESC (Biobanco de Dentes Humanos da Faculdade do Oeste de Santa Catarina - Joa^aba) to:

1. **Cite in all publications** the number of teeth used in the work and that they originated from the BDH/UNOESC.
2. **Send a copy of** the published work(s) in which the BDH/UNOESC is mentioned.

Joa^aba, 20

____
Signature of applicant

Prof^s _______________________________
Coordinator of the BDH/UNOESC

ANNEX VI

1-DECLARATION **TO THE RESEARCH ETHICS COMMITTEE**

For the purposes of evaluation by the Research Ethics Committee (CEP) of this institution, the Human Tooth Bank of UNOESC is once again committed to helping researchers carry out their projects.

Therefore, following approval by the CEP, our contribution will consist of offering (tooth group number) _______________ for the execution of the research work entitled: "

____

" to be carried out by (author(s)) __ and guided by.

Joa^aba, 20.

_______________________________ Coordinator
of the BDH/UNOESC

ANNEX VII
TERM OF CONCESSION

I, an undergraduate student in the dentistry course at UNOESC, bearer of registration number _______________ residing in _______________________________,

neighborhood, city, UF, zip code, telephone number, hereby grant tooth(s) to the UNOESC Human Teeth Biobank, on the understanding that they will be used by undergraduate and postgraduate students at this Faculty for study and research. The research must have been previously approved by the HUST Research Ethics Committee.

Origin of the teeth:

Joa^aba, 20 _______________________________ .

____

Signature

2-DECLARATION TO THE RESEARCH ETHICS COMMITTEE FOR NEW RESEARCH.

For the purposes of evaluation by the Research Ethics Committee (CEP) of this institution, the UNOESC Human Teeth Biobank undertakes to inform the CEP whenever new research is started using the same tooth under our concession.

Therefore, after approval by the CEP, our contribution will consist of offering (number of group of teeth) _____________________ for the execution of the entitled research work:
"" to be realized by (author(s))
____ and guided by

Joa^aba, 20 .

____
BDH General Coordinator

TERM OF CONCESSION OF HUMAN TEETH
DENTAL SURGEON

I, , Dental Surgeon, registered with the CRO, bearer of the CPF with office located in the neighborhood, city, UF, zip code, telephone, grant teeth to the BIOBANCO
OF HUMAN TEETH OF THE COURSE OF ODONTOLOGY OF THE UNIVERSITY OF THE WEST OF SANTA CATARINA - UNOESC, declaring that these teeth were extracted by therapeutic indication, whose histories are part of the medical records of the patients from whom they originate, filed under my responsibility, I declare that I am delivering together with the teeth the ICF and consent form signed by the patients. Joa^aba, of 20.

____ Signature

ANNEX VIII
INTERNAL CONTROL SHEET

Number:
Name:RG:
Address:Neighborhood:
Zip code:City:State:
Fone (res):Celular :Consultorio:
e-mail: _____________________________
COURSE:
Graduate - Current class:Graduate - Department :
Specialized - area :Other - please specify:

Relevant comments :

Teeth donated to the BDH

Date/Phase	Quantity	Discipline	Condition	Signature

Teeth lent by the BDH.				
Date/Phase	Quantity	Discipline	Condition	Signature
Teeth returned to the BDH.				
Date/Phase	Quantity	Discipline	Condition	Signature

To use the tooth biobank
Record number: _________________________ bookpage ____________

ANNEX IX

A

NATIONAL RESEARCH ETHICS COMMISSION - CONEP. MINISTRY OF HEALTH
BRASILIA - DF

TERM OF INSTITUTIONAL RESPONSIBILITY (TRI)

The Universidade do Oeste de Santa Catarina - Unoesc, maintained by the Fundado Universidade do Oeste de Santa Catarina - Funoesc, represented by the Rector Professor Aristides Cimadon, holder of RG 3.620.711 SSP/SC, registered with the CPF under[0] 180.891.009-53, hereby declares its technical and financial responsibility for setting up and maintaining the Human Teeth Biobank (BDH) of the Universidade do Oeste de Santa Catarina - UNOESC, classified as a Biobank, in order to request its regularization and accreditation before the National Research Ethics Commission (CONEP/MS), taking into account National Health Council Resolution No. 441 of May 12, 2011 and Ministry of Health Ordinance No. 2,201 of September 14, 2011.

It also states that Unoesc's Human Teeth Biobank (BDH) complies with institutional regulations for the development of teaching, research and extension, contributing to regional development.

Joacaba/SC, August 05, 2016.

Rector of the university.

ANNEX X

TERM OF RESPONSIBILITY FOR MANAGEMENT

We hereby declare that we are responsible for the management of the Human Teeth Biobank (BDH) of the Universidade do Oeste de Santa Catarina - and we are aware of the legal charges mentioned by the Resolution of the National Health Council no.[0] 441, of May 12, 2011 and the Ministry of Health Ordinance no. 2.201, of September 14, 2011.

We also declare that the Unoesc Biobanco has a set of practices, equipment and facilities aimed at human health care and the development of teaching, research and extension in higher education.

Joa^aba/SC, January 16, 2017.

Prof.[1] . Bruna Eliza DeDea
Coordinator of the Dentistry Course Unoesc/Joa^aba
CPF: 05310329-80
Contact: (49) 999178881 e-mail:bruna.dedea@unoesc.edu.br

Prof.ª Léa Maria Franceschi Dallanora,
General Coordinator of the BDH
CPF: 496072439-00
Contact: (49) 991042226 e-mail: lea.dallanora@unoesc.edu.br
Prof. Acir José Dirschnabel;
Responsible for capturing teeth
CPF:02460301944
Contact: (41) 99813612 e-mail: acir.dirschnabel@unoesc.edu.br
Prof. Fábio José Dallanora;
Responsible for Microbiological Control
CPF:38696487915
Contact: (49) 988311454 e-mail: fabio.dallanora@unoesc.edu.br

ANNEX XI

TRANSFER OF BIOLOGICAL MATERIAL

The Material Transfer Agreement (TTM) was established to control the non-commercial exchange of biological material existing *in situ, in* the national territory, on the continental shelf and exclusive economic zone, kept in *ex situ* conditions, destined for biological institutions or collections based abroad, based on the following premises:

The recognition that the non-commercial exchange of biological material between collections or research institutions in the biological and related areas is fundamental for the advancement of knowledge about Brazilian biodiversity;

The need to guarantee compliance with the provisions of the Convention on International Trade in Endangered Species of Wild Flora and Fauna (CITES) and the Convention on Biological Diversity (CBD), in particular national sovereignty over its biological diversity.

№ OF TTM/ (year)
Sending institution: UNIVERSITY OF WESTERN SANTA CATARINA
CNPJ: 84.592.369/0001-20
Address: Rua GETULIO VARGAS 2125 Telephone- 55 49 35512242
Name of curator: Léa Maria Franceschi Dallanora
Identification Document : CPF 49607243900
Position of curator: Biobank Coordinator
Recipient institution or collection:
Address:
Name of the representative of the receiving institution or collection:
Identity document (type, number and issuing body):
Position of the representative of the receiving institution:

The signatory iiistiUicies, qualified above, through their representatives, in view of the provisions of CITES and CBD, undertake to use the biological material transferred between them in accordance with the following conditions:

1. The biological material received must be used by the recipient institution or college exclusively for the development of scientific research with no potential for economic use.

2. If there is any interest in starting a bioprospecting or technological development

activity, or in applying for a patent using the biological material sent on the basis of this Agreement, the receiving institution is obliged to notify the sending institution and the latter the Genetic Heritage Management Council (CGEN).

3. It is forbidden to start the activities mentioned in the previous item without observing the provisions of current legislation, in particular, obtaining specific authorizations from CGEN.

4. Biological material shipped on the basis of this TTM will only be passed on to third parties by the receiving organization once a new TTM has been signed between the original sending organization and the new receiving organization.

5. The recipient institution that receives the biological material must respect the terms of the TTM and will not be considered the provider of the material received.

6. Any publication resulting from the use or study of the biological material sent must expressly acknowledge the origin of the material and credit the sending institution, and a copy of the publication must be sent to the sending institution.

7. The signatory institutions or collections shall collaborate on the basis of mutually agreed terms for the training and transfer of technology in order to promote the conservation and sustainable use of biological diversity.

8. It is the sole responsibility of the sending institution or collection to identify and properly package the material, and to carry out the shipping procedures in accordance with the regulations pertaining to the biological risk classification and containment of the organism or material to be transferred, observing the recommendations of the competent bodies, international standards and specific legislation of the recipient country.

9.		The recipient institution undertakes to:

a) not claim, on its own behalf or on behalf of third parties, any form of intellectual property over all or part of the biological material transferred under these Terms.

b) inform the sending institution or collection, in writing, of any adverse effect that may have occurred during the handling of the biological material covered by this Agreement.

10. The place of jurisdiction for the settlement of disputes between the institutions or collections involved in this TTM shall be the seat of the sending institution.

11. The commitments relating to the material transferred by means of this Agreement remain valid for an indefinite period, regardless of their renewal.

In agreement with all the terms set out above, the representatives of the recipient institution or collection and the sender institution or collection sign this Agreement in two copies of equal content and form, for one legal purpose only.

Place and date:_______________________________________

Representative of the receiving institution:

____

Institution representative

sender: _______________________________________

ANNEX XII

LETTER OF COMMUNICATION TO THE CONSENTING PARTY FOR SUBSEQUENT DISPOSAL OF THE BIOLOGICAL MATERIAL.

BIOBANK DECLARATION

Dear Sir, We would like to inform you that your concession of tooth number(s) to the UNOESC Biobanks, which took place on the date of
.... after being used   in research, it will no longer be used and will be disposed of as biological material in accordance with CNS Resolution No.^{0} 441 of 2011, items 7 and 8; MS Ordinance No.^{0} 2.201 of 2011, Sole

Paragraph. If the SR. wishes to remove the waste from his concession, it will be at his disposal until the date   of the withdrawal.
after this date it will be sent and collected by the team that collects the dental waste at UNOESC.
Without further ado, we look forward to your reply. Sincerely.
.... Joa^abade20 ....

____
General coordinator of the BDH

5.2 OPERATIONAL PROCEDURES (SOPs)
5.3 1 How to draw up the BDH's Standard Operating Procedures.

- The purpose of UNOESC's human teeth biobank is to correctly and sterilely store the dental elements that are awarded, which will then be sent to a specific destination.
- The preparation of teeth arriving at the BDH includes the stages of handling, selection, storage and disinfection and/or sterilization.
- It is the BDH's responsibility to ensure that the infection caused by the indiscriminate handling of extracted teeth is eliminated. For a BDH to function properly, it is essential to have strict control of its internal procedures, which include sorting and stocking teeth, as well as registering and filing the records of consenters or beneficiaries.
- The BHD's aim with regard to the teeth collected is to meet scientific needs by providing human teeth for research.

5.2.2 Captured from dental elements

The teeth stored in UNOESC's Biobank of human teeth come from grants, collected from private clinics, health centers and the institution's dental clinics. Teeth are also collected by students in their communities through grants from patients.

- Priority must be given to the legality of the origin of the captured teeth
- In cases where one or more teeth are to be extracted from a patient, the patient should be asked if he or she agrees to have the teeth donated and should be informed through the ICF as to where the teeth will go and for what purpose they will be used. If they agree, they should be asked to sign the Informed Consent Form.
- Another way of collecting teeth is from dentists who have teeth. In this case, the TCLE and the Term of Granting of Human Teeth from Dental Surgeons are used, where the professional will be granting all the teeth that are stored in his or her office, taking responsibility for their origin. If the DC does not have an ICF for the tooth, it will be sent to the tooth bank and used for teaching purposes.

5.2.3 Transportation (receiving and sending dental elements)

> Research activities.

The teeth will be delivered upon request in the appropriate term (TTMB) for activities carried out in research at UNOESC and/or another educational institution that is a partner in research.

5.2.4 Cleaning, preparation and selection of incoming teeth.

> Teeth should be cleaned using distilled water and curettes to scrape and remove any organic dendrites.

> - Teeth must be selected in order to separate healthy, decayed, restored and discarded teeth (unable to be used for research).

5.2.5 Packaging, sterilization and storage.

> When we receive the teeth, we sterilize them on surgical-grade paper to reduce the bacterial flora.

> The tooth must then be cleaned.

> Once the teeth have been cleaned, they are packed in glass jars, filled with distilled water, the glass is recapped and sterilized.

> Storage should be done in a specific cupboard when the vials do not show any signs of contamination.

5.2.6 Loan and disposal of dental elements

5.2.6.1. Loans are made when a researcher needs such teeth and doesn't have them, he or she makes a request to the Human Teeth Biobank of the Universidade do Oeste de Santa Catarina, fulfilling all the requirements demanded by the coordinators of the Human Teeth Biobank.

5.2.6.2. -After approval by the CEPs of the institutions involved and with all the paperwork completed in accordance with the requirements of the BDH, the teeth will be sent to the researcher together with the Term of transfer of biological material (duly completed).

5.2.6.3. - In principle, all the material collected will be used for research until it is finished, but if it is necessary to discard it, this is done when the BDH team concludes that the tooth is no longer suitable for research. This disposal is carried out in accordance with CNS Resolution n^0 441 of 2011, items 7 and 8; MS Ordinance n^0 2.201 of 2011, Sole Paragraph, so at this point the consenter will be informed about the loss, alteration or destruction of their biological samples, as well as about the closure or transfer of biological material between biobanks, when applicable, being discarded and collected by the team that collects the dental waste from UNOESC.

5.2.7 Microbiological quality control.

Control of the microbiota is carried out according to the general bacteriological technique since the main objective is to avoid the spread and/or cross-contamination by microorganisms. The dental elements come from extractions carried out at the University's dental clinics, health centers and private practices in the region. When these teeth are received "in natura", biosafety procedures are initiated to eliminate microorganisms from the initial care site, interrupting the chain of cross-transmission.

- The first procedure is to autoclave the dental elements for sterilization and then store them in a safe, contaminant-free place.
- The procedures for controlling microbiology start as soon as these items are received, with the use of PPE, cleaning, packaging and sterilizing them.

The materials used, such as the autoclave, are also periodically maintained and cleaned according to university protocol.

5.2.8 Selection of trainees.

Monitors (trainees) are selected by means of an application form which is sent by the dentistry course secretary when the application period opens, together with the public notice. The form must be duly filled in with the student's registration details and available timetables, and a copy of the student's transcript must be attached for analysis and subsequent submission to the secretary's office.

When the monitors are informed of their choice, they sign a monitoring contract: UNIVERSIDADE DO OESTE DE SANTA CATARINA - UNOESC, accredited by the

Presidential Decree of August 14, 1996, qualified as a Community Institution of Higher Education - ICES, under the terms of Law n^0 12.881/13 and Portaria n^0 634, of October 30, 2014, maintained by FUNDAQÁO UNIVERSIDADE DO OESTE DE SANTA CATARINA - FUNOESC, created by Municipal Law 545/68 and a non-profit private law structure, registered with the CNPJ under 84.592.369/0001-20, with headquarters at Rua Getúlio Vargas, 2125, CEP 89.600-000, Bairro Flor da Serra, Joacaba/SC, by its legal representative. In this contract, the clauses make clear the functions and obligations of the monitors, as well as the hours and periods, that these activities will not be remunerated and that they will be under the guidance of the course coordinator and also, in the Human Teeth Biobanks, of the teacher responsible.

Monitors must take part in drawing up and implementing the activities set out in the action plan drawn up by the members of the BDH, supervised and guided by the teacher in charge and the course coordinator. Involvement in all activities, meetings, responsibility and commitment to excellence must always be respected.

ANNEX XIII
ARTICLES ABOUT THE BDH

ARTICLE 1:

IMPLEMENTATION OF THE HUMAN TEETH BANK - BDH OF THE
DENTISTRY COURSE AT
THE UNIVERSITY OF WESTERN SANTA CATARINA

Carem Zanatta[*]
Thaíse Pródocimo [*][1]
Lea Maria Fransceschi Dallanora [2][†][‡]

SUMMARY

Human tooth banks are an important didactic, scientific and clinical tool that is increasingly present in Brazilian dental courses. At the Unoesc Dentistry Course, it began operating on March 17, 2011. Its purpose was to organize and facilitate the collection, storage and donation of teeth, formalizing their origin and destination and creating ideal conditions for the use of these organs. Thus, this work seeks to demonstrate how the implementation of the BDH at Unoesc took place, from the physical adequacy project, structuring for collection, storage and donation, document organization, functionality and bureaucratic facts to the start of its activities.
Keywords: Human tooth bank. Structuring a DBH. Organizing and Managing. Storing Human Teeth.

INTRODUCTION

The implementation of the Human Tooth Bank (HDB) in the Dentistry Course at Unoesc aims to meet the need for human teeth in the learning process of undergraduate and postgraduate dentists. Human teeth are used in pre-clinical laboratory activities for undergraduates and postgraduates and are also used in *in vitro* research for course final papers. This is because the Ethics and Research Committees (CEP) require that the origin of the teeth used in such research be detailed for project approval (NASSIF et al., 2003).

The Unoesc Human Tooth Bank was structured in accordance with Research Project No. 1149/09, Process No. 1255/10 and Resolution No. 01/CG/ll, respecting the Institution's statutes. It has its own internal regulations, a physical space duly equipped for the disinfection and storage of dental elements, in accordance with university policy and the economic reality of the region in which it is located. In order for the BDH to operate perfectly, it has a protocol for receiving donations, requesting and using permanent and deciduous human teeth.

The Tooth Bank is organized to facilitate the collection and donation or loan of teeth, taking care of their origin, which must have the consent of the donor, as well as their destination, creating ideal conditions for the use of these organs in accordance with the Brazilian Transplant Law (Law n. 9,434, of February 4, 1997) and with the National Health Council (Resolution n. 196, of October 10, 1996) (BRASIL, 1996, 1997; FERREIRA et al., 2003).

In order to facilitate the necessary implementation of the BDHs, there should be more information and guidance on the mechanisms of their implementation, including aspects such as structure, organization, functionality, tooth collection and biosafety. In addition, the aim is to describe the situation of the dental teaching institutions in the state of Santa Catarina with regard to the existence of BDHs. Here, we will discuss

---

[*]Dental Surgeon, graduated from the Universidade do Oeste de Santa Catarina; Rúa Cel. Fagundes, 128, Bairro Santo Antonio, 89620-000, Campos Novos, SC; E-mail: carem zanatta@hotmail.com.

[†]Dental Surgeon, graduated from the University of the West of Santa Catarina. Rúa, SC; E-mail

[‡] Master Dental Surgeon, specialist in University of   the West of Santa Catarina; Rúa Cel. , n. , Neighborhood , 89620 000, Campos Novos, SC; E-mail

the functions that a DBH can perform and the way in which the Human Tooth Bank of the Unoesc Dentistry Course is currently organized and functioning.

MATERIAL AND METHODS

This is a descriptive exploratory study.

The following instruments were used to collect the information:

a) Open interview with the team responsible;
b) Documentary analysis (BDH implementation project);
c) Documentary analysis - ethics committee opinion, BDH statute and Unoesc regulations;
d) Observing everyday life;
e) Review of the relevant literature;
f) Survey of other BHD experiences.

RESULTS AND DISCUSSION

The Tooth Bank is a promising investment for the dental health area, and can bring benefits to the population, however, it is essential to collaborate in the safe handling for learning, research and technological innovations that make use of human teeth (MOREIRA et al., 2009). With this in mind, the University of Western Santa Catarina (Unoesc) has invested in BDH as a means of benefiting the public and avoiding cross-contamination between academics, teachers and even the public.

The creation of tooth banks in Brazilian Dental Teaching Institutions should be the best way to comply with current legislation on research involving human beings (BRASIL, 1996). At Unoesc, the BDH was made official in March 2011, in accordance with Resolution No. 01/CG/11, which commenced its activities, such as collecting dental organs, cleaning and storing them.

There is not enough information and data available on how to organize and use tooth banks ethically and rationally, and which dental schools maintain them, or even intend to create them (BEGOSSO et al., 2001). Unoesc's DBH was developed using Professor Jose Carlos Imparato's book as a model, which has been a guide for the implementation of many DBHs, as he was the forerunner in the creation of this body within dentistry.

One of the most important reasons for the approval of the implementation of the BDH at Unoesc by the Management Council was the fact reported by Pinto et al. (2009), where the CEP does not accept research involving human teeth without proven origin. In addition, the Organ Transplant Law (BRASIL, 1997) states that it is a crime to handle organs or parts of organs without documenting their origin and donating them. Therefore, in view of the large number of research projects carried out with dental elements by teachers and academics, the board of the institution decided that the BDH should be set up.

It was also observed that the main sources of demand for and collection of teeth were dental practices, health centers and hospitals (ZUCCO et al., 2006). When the BDH was set up at Unoesc, the collection, which today has around 10,121 teeth, was mainly donated by academics, dentists and teachers who gave their private collections.

The creation of the DBH requires several stages; starting with the project to be drawn up for approval, then the statute or regulation, depending on the institution to which the tooth bank is linked, and must always follow Anvisa standards (IMPARATO et al., 2003). At Unoesc, the implementation process also went through several stages, starting with the creation project. Once approved, it was possible to start adapting the physical space, which was equipped according to the instructions described in the book *Banco de Dentes Humanos,* by Jose Carlos Pettorossi Imparato e Colaboradores, and the Anvisa instructions (IMPARATO et al., 2003). Secondly, the tooth donations were catalogued, cleaned and packaged and, finally, their legalization was studied, where the Unoesc BDH regulations were drawn up, following the laws and statutes of the Institution.

A functioning DBH must have regulations or statutes specifying all the documents needed for it to function properly, and these regulations must state who is responsible for the DBH (NASSIF et al., 2003). In the case of the BDH at Unoesc, there are regulations; this is because Unoesc believes that the tooth bank is an extension of the Dentistry Course and is governed by it, rather than a separate body with a statute. According to Article 3 of the regulations, the BDH has a general coordinator, a position held by the course coordinator, and an auxiliary coordinator, a course lecturer who is responsible for the tooth bank, as well as three trainees who are responsible for receiving, cleaning and storing the bank's teeth.

And according to Article 9 of the regulation, the Unoesc tooth bank has its own book, with numbered pages, with opening and closing terms initialed by the competent health authority, which is used to register donor patients and their identity number, and another book with the same characteristics for registering patients who receive donated teeth, or requesting professors.

The BDH at Unoesc, according to the architectural plan, has a usable physical area of $39m^2$, which is larger than the minimum stipulated in Professor Imparato's book. Photograph 1 of the BDH shows the reception room, where the administrative room is located, consisting of a microcomputer, filing cabinet, fax, telephone, desks, cupboards and other office materials.

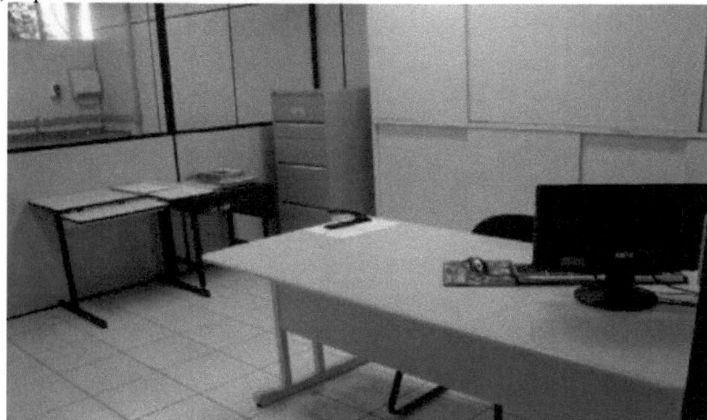

Photograph 1: Reception room of the Unoesc BDH Source: the authors.

Photo 2 shows the BDH room, with a bench for sorting and cleaning teeth, sinks and cupboards, and an autoclave for sterilizing teeth. In this room there are refrigerators for storing the teeth, which is in line with current health surveillance standards, which state that for the BDH to function properly, a laboratory and a support room are necessary. According to Nassif et al. (2003), moist heat without a drying process is the best way of sterilizing teeth (largely supported by scientific research) and does not significantly alter the physical and chemical properties of the tooth. According to Imparato et al. (2003), teeth should be preserved in liquid to remain hydrated and should also be stored under refrigeration.

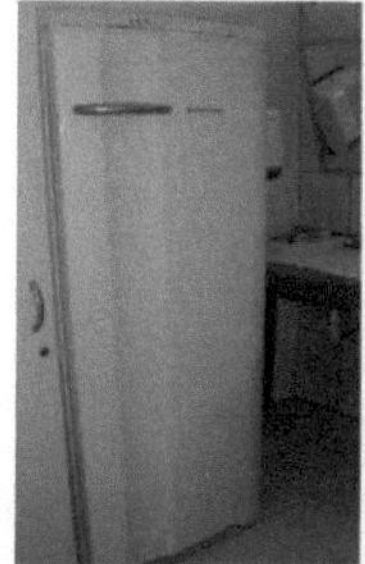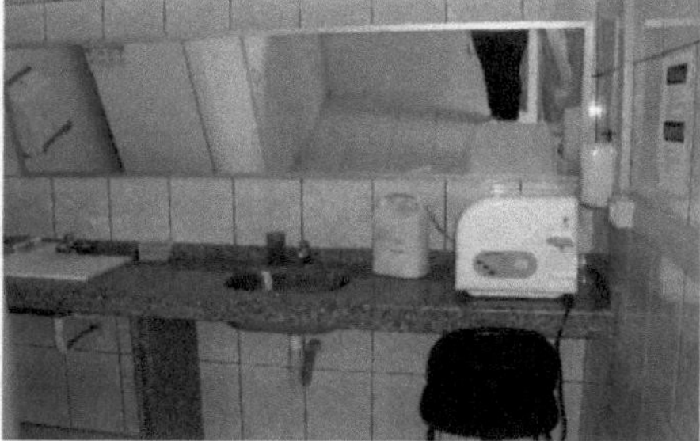

Photo 2: Room with the bench for selecting and cleaning teeth, an autoclave and a fridge for storing teeth. Source: the authors.

According to Ferreira et al. (2003), the teeth in the DBH must be of proven origin, by means of a donation form. The BDH must be organized and have careful functionality so that everything can be carried out within the rules established by the institution's regulations, not forgetting the Free and Informed Consent document for using the teeth and signed by the individual donor. At Unoesc's BDH, donations are received by means of a Donation Form, with one type of form for each situation, an individual one for the donor of their tooth, a specific one for deciduous teeth, where the parents or guardians are the donors, specific terms for private dental surgeons' collections, specific terms for health departments and the like.

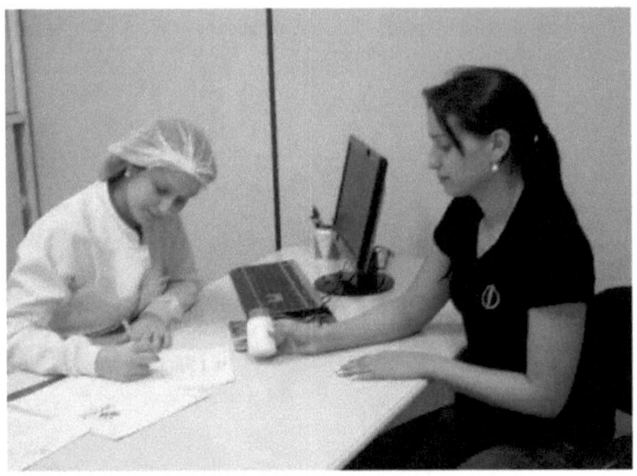

Photo 3: Intern at the Unoesc BDH receiving the teeth Source: the authors.

The BDHs linked to dental courses reduce the risk of cross-infection due to incorrect handling of dental organs and organize the supply of these elements to undergraduate and postgraduate students (POLETTO et al., 2010).

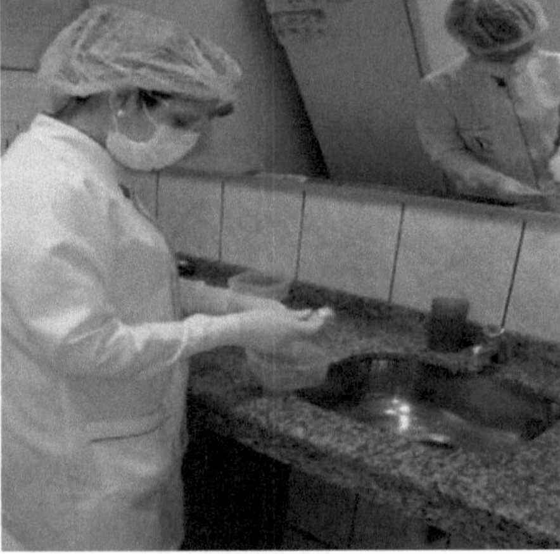

Photo 4: Trainee from the BDH brushing her teeth. Source: the authors.

Thus, the BDH at Unoesc receives the donated dental element, which, after being catalogued, is cleaned with soap and water; caries lesions, calculus and bone debris are then removed by scraping the surface with curettes, ultrasound devices and using a high/low speed motor. They are then separated into groups according to their anatomy and position in the oral cavity, and then placed in an appropriate, sterilized package, and finally stored in distilled water, which is changed weekly.

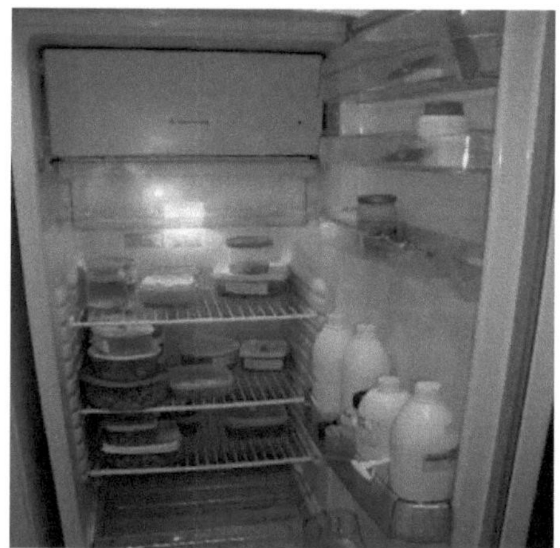
Photo 5: Teeth stored in the fridge with distilled water Source: the authors.

At Unoesc's BDH, according to its regulations, teeth for teaching purposes are only sterilized immediately before being delivered to the requesting students, wrapped in gauze, in packaging suitable for autoclaving. The teeth can be separated according to the needs of each discipline,

Teeth for research purposes, following the new provisions of the Brazilian Transplant Law, must be stored individually in distilled water and properly identified and cataloged. The water must be changed weekly.

In order to borrow the teeth, undergraduates must sign a registration form and undertake to return them at the end of the current semester. The number and type of teeth loaned to each student is agreed between the Human Teeth Bank and the head of the requesting department. For scientific research, researchers interested in acquiring teeth should contact the Tooth Bank to check availability. The Tooth Bank provides the researcher with a letter for submission to the Ethics Committee. After approval by the Research Ethics Committee, the teeth are released to the researcher (IMPARATO et al., 2003). According to the procedures of the Unoesc Human Tooth Bank, the loan of teeth for clinical and therapeutic purposes will be subject to a prior request from the registered dental surgeon and the patient's free and informed consent; the Human Tooth Bank will be responsible for sterilizing and storing the tooth selected for biological restoration.

According to Avelar et al. (2009), it is important to emphasize that when teeth are used for bonding, it is essential to sterilize the teeth using the moist heat technique. In addition, as with any clinical procedure, the patient must be informed about the treatment options; then, they or their legal guardian, in the case of minors, must authorize the procedure. At Unoesc, no research has yet been carried out using deciduous or permanent BDH teeth clinically.

For Ulson and Imparato (2008), in the clinical case they reported of coronary destruction of deciduous molars due to caries, in which the technique of bonding dental fragments that were part of the tooth bank was used after a four-year period of monitoring the restorations, they concluded that the technique is an alternative for oral rehabilitation in cases of loss of dental structure. Unoesc, despite having deciduous teeth in its collection, has not yet carried out any research in the area of paediatric dentistry and long-term follow-up, as the BDH began its activities only a short time ago; with the increase in publicity and students' knowledge of its usefulness, there will still be a lot of research to be carried out.

According to Zucco et al. (2006), surprisingly, during their research they found that the students were aware of what the tooth bank was; however, there was a great deal of resistance on the part of the students when it came to donating teeth to the bank; this may have been due to a lack of knowledge about the bank's activities and the rules of procedure regarding the donation and removal of dental elements. To date, the BDH at Unoesc has received 186 teeth extracted in the course's clinics, 890 donated by course teachers and students, 1,980 donated by health departments in other municipalities, 6,185 teeth from dentistry and endodontics courses and around 500 donated by the course's anatomy laboratory. It has already lent around 400 teeth for research by academics (BDH-UNOESC, 2011).

It is understood that it takes some time for the culture of valuing the tooth as an organ to be formed; therefore, it is essential that dental schools include information on this subject in their curricula and that more scientific studies are developed (PINTO et al., 2009).

However, it is not only important for the process of setting up the BDH in universities to be exposed, but it is also necessary for academics themselves to publicize it to society, in order to make people aware that donating teeth to the BDH will benefit society, academics, research and everyone who needs procedures such as biological restorations. The BDH at Unoesc was publicized through students presenting their work at the Academic Week held for the Dentistry Course, also by teachers in the classroom and to the scientific community and society through the spoken media: Unoesc Joanaba radio and Catarinense radio; through interviews and the written media, through local newspapers.

CONCLUSION

This study shows how the BDH at Unoesc was set up, how it was organized and how it is working and using its collection, demonstrating its importance in the scenario of dentistry courses, especially at Unoesc. The organization of the collection and its documentation provides the BDH with optimum functionality, as we observed through this research. We observed through the documentary archives that since the BDH was set up, our academics have used dental elements from the BDH in their pre-clinical activities and that the research carried out has also used teeth from this same source, and even teeth from the BDH have not been used as biological restorations because there is still a need for more research in this area. Thus, we can say that the BDH is installed, duly documented and fully operational, in accordance with current Anvisa standards and within the norms of the Unoesc Statute.

ESTABLISHMENT OF THE BANK OF HUMAN TEETH-BDH COURSE OF DENTISTRY UNIVERSITY OF THE WEST OF ST CATHERINE

ABSTRACT

The Banks of Human Teeth are an important educational, scientific and clinical tool that is increasingly present in the Brazilian of Dentistry coursers. In the Dentistry course of the UNOESC the Bank of Human Teeth began operating on March 17, 2011. Its implementation had the purpose to organize and facilitate the capture, storage and donation of the teeth, formalizing its source and destination providing ideal conditions for the use of this organ. So, we demonstrated how the implantation of the BHT of the UNOESC occurred from the physical adequacy of the project, organization to capture, storage and donation, organization of documents, functionality and the bureaucracy to the beginning of its activities.

Keywords: Banks of Human Teeth. Organization the BHT. Organization and Administration. Storage of Human Teeth.

REFERENCES

NATIONAL HEALTH SURVEILLANCE AGENCY. **Dental services**: risk prevention and control. Brasilia, DF: 2006. Available at: <http://www.anvisa.gov.br/servicosaude/manuais /manual_odonto.pdf>. Accessed on: September 7, 2011.

AVELAR, Felipe Morando et al. Homogenous bonding of a tooth fragment in a permanent maxillary central incisor - clinical case report. **RFO**, v. 14,n. 1, p. 66-70, Jan./Apr. 2009. .

BEGOSSO, M. P.; IMPARATO, J. C. P.; DUARTE, D. A. Current status of the organization of human tooth banks in dental schools in Brazil.
RPGRev. Pós Grad., v. 8,n.1, 23-28,jan./mar. 2001.

BRASIL. Resoluto n. 196, de16de outubro de 1996. **Diario Oficial da Umao**, October 16, 1996. Available at: <www.conselho.saude.gov.br>. Accessed on: October 6, 2011.

BRAZIL. Law n. 9.434, of February 4, 1997. Provides for the Removal of Organs, Tissues and Parts of the Human Body for Transplant and Treatment Purposes and other Provisions. **Diario Oficial [da] República Federativa do** Brasil, Brasilia, DF, Feb. 5, 1997. Available at:
http://www6.senado.gov.br/legislacao/ListaTextoIntegral.action7idM23711>. Accessed on: Feb. 5, 2011.

FEDERAL COUNCIL OF DENTISTRY. List of Colleges in the State of Santa Catarina. Available at: <http://odontologika.uol.com.br/fac_santacatarina.htm>. Accessed on: October 5, 2011.

IMPARATO, Jose Carlos Pettorossi et al. **Banco de Dentes Humanos**. Curitiba: Ed. Maio, Curitiba, 2003.

MOREIRA,L. et al. Banco de Dentes Humanos para o Ensino e Pesquisa em Odontologia. **Rev. Fac. Odontol.**, Porto Alegre, v. 50, n. 1, p. 34-37, jan./abr., 2009.

NASSIF, A. C. S. et al. Structuring a Human Tooth Bank. **Pesq. Odontol. Bras.**, Sao Paulo, v. 17, p. 70-74, May 2003.

PINTO, L. S. et al. Popular, Academic and Professional Knowledge about the Human Tooth Bank. **Pesq. Bras. Odontoped. Clin. Integr.**, Joao Pessoa, v. 9,n. 1, p. 101-106, Jan./Apr. 2009.

POLETTO, M. M. et al. Human Tooth Bank: Socio-Cultural Profile of a Group of Donors. **RGO**, Porto Alegre, v. 58,n. 1, p. 91-94, Jan./Mar. 2010.

ULSON , Raquel Cristina Barbosa, IMPARATO, Jose Carlos Pettorossi. Oral Rehabilitation through

Fragment Bonding in Deciduous Teeth. **Publ. UEPG Ci. Biol. Saúde**, Ponta Grossa, v. 14,n. 1, p. 23-28, Mar. 2008.

ZUCCO, Debora et al. Evaluation of the Level of Knowledge of UNIVILLE Dentistry Course Students on the Utilization of Extracted Teeth in the

Graduate and Tooth Bank. **Revista Sul-Brasileira de Odontologia**, v. 3,n. 1,p. 55, 2006.

ARTICLE 2:

RECOGNIZING THE IMPORTANCE OF THE TOOTH AS A HUMAN ORGAN

RECOGNITION OF THE IMPORTANCE OF TOOTH AS A HUMAN BODY

SUMMARY

The aim of this article was to assess knowledge about ethics, organ donation, the importance of valuing the tooth as an organ, knowledge of the existence of a human tooth bank (HDB) among academics, dental professionals and lay people, and to check whether these groups have knowledge about the correct destination of dental elements and root remains after their extraction. To carry out the study, a questionnaire with multiple-choice questions was drawn up and 180 individuals (60 dental surgeons, 60 dental academics and 60 lay people) were interviewed in the Midwest region of Santa Catarina. Based on the interviews, it was observed that the majority of those interviewed were in favor of organ donation. With regard to the dental element, 89.8% of academics, 50.9% of laypeople and the vast majority of dentists (98.3%) consider the tooth to be a human organ, and all three groups would use the teeth stored in a BHD as restorative material. Regarding what is done with extracted teeth, 11.7% of laypeople, 40% of academics and 65% of professionals are aware that these organs should be sent and stored in BHDs. Based on the results, it can be concluded that the population is aware of and in favour of organ donation, that teeth are recognized as organs of the human body among academics and dentists, and that the lay population still needs further clarification about teeth being organs and the destination of these organs after extraction. As a result, the dental organ deserves legal, bioethical and biosafety recognition, as well as proper storage.

KEYWORDS: Tooth; Donation; Ethics; Organ.

ABSTRACT

This article focused on evaluating the knowledge about ethics, organ donation, the importance of valuing the tooth as an organ, the knowledge of the existence of a bank of human teeth (BHT) among academics, dental professionals and laypersons, and verify that these groups have the correct knowledge about the destination that should be given to the teeth and root fragments after extraction. To develop the study a questionnaire was designed with multiple choice questions, being interviewed 180 people (60 dentists, 60 dental students and 60 laymen), in the region of Midwest Catarinense. Based on the interviews, it can be noted that most of the target audience is in favor of organ donation. Concerning the dental element, 89.8% of the students, 50.9% of the laity and the vast majority of dentists (98.3%) believe the tooth a human organ, however the three groups would use their teeth stored in a BHT as a restorative material. Regarding what is done with the extracted teeth, 11.7% of the laity, 40% of students and 65% of professionals aware that these bodies should be routed and stored in BHT's. We can conclude then that the teeth are recognized as human body organs among dentists and dental students and the lay population that need further clarification on what is done with the teeth after extraction, therefore the dental organ deserves legal recognition, bioethics, biosecurity and proper storage.

KEYWORDS: Tooth; Donation; Ethics; Organ.

1. INTRODUCTION

The recognition of the dental element is a factor that is often overlooked by most dentists and by some professionals involved in scientific research, who use large quantities of human teeth in their work, disregarding the ethical, legal, cultural and social aspects of the dental organ.[1]

In addition to the importance of knowing where extracted human teeth come from and how they are used in the teaching and learning process, another important issue is knowing which decontamination and storage procedures are being used in accordance with biosafety standards.[2]

Knowing the origin of the dental organ makes it possible to add social value to the donated organ, generating greater commitment to the processes and results in all lines of dental research.[3]

In vitro studies on human teeth make a great contribution to the teaching of different areas of dentistry, as they enable techniques to be evaluated, materials to be tested and new methods and products to be developed, with a view to improving the quality of dental services provided to the population.[4]

The importance of recognizing the tooth as an organ is also to prevent the spread of disease, as it is known that every organ in the human body is a source of pathogens for humans. Micro-organisms found in extracted teeth or teeth in the oral cavity can cause and transmit infectious diseases. Some pathogens can survive for a long time on extracted teeth, enabling cross-contamination and various infections.

Therefore, the existence of a differentiated institution, exclusively concerned with dental organs, is justified by legal, bioethical, cultural and social reasons.[1] The purpose of Human Tooth Banks (HDBs) is to reduce the risk of cross-infections arising from the incorrect handling of dental organs, organize the supply of these elements for loan and, consequently, eliminate the illegal trade in teeth[4] , as well as to raise awareness among individuals about the importance of teeth as organs and their relationship with general health, disseminating information about their use in scientific research and treatment.[6]

The Human Tooth Bank is concerned with the origin and destination of extracted teeth. In 1997, the Transplant Law was created in Brazil (Law 9.434 of 04/02/1997), in which teeth became recognized as organs. This law provides for a penalty of three to eight years in prison and a fine for anyone who removes organs, tissues and parts of the human body from unidentified people *post-mortem*.[7] The Penal Code also provides for a penalty of one to three years' imprisonment for those who violate graves (Article 210), and the National Health Council requires the subjects to provide Terms of Free and Informed Consent as a form of "respect for human dignity".[8] The tooth, like any other organ of the human body, can only be donated with the consent of the patient or guardian, which is expressed to the Human Tooth Bank through a Free and Informed Consent Form. Therefore, the implementation of the Human Tooth Bank in Dental Teaching Institutions seems to be the best way to comply with current legislation regarding research involving human beings and the removal of organs, tissues and parts of the human body for treatment purposes.[9] Therefore, the donor's authorization is required for the use of teeth. In view of the establishment of the BDH as a place to store these elements, it seeks to facilitate the collection, donation or loan of teeth to those who need the institution's services.

The purpose of this study was to assess knowledge about ethics, organ donation, the importance of valuing the tooth as an organ and the existence of a human tooth bank among academics, dental professionals and lay people.

2. MATERIALSANDMETHODS

The study in question adopts a predominantly quantitative research approach, as it uses standardized data that allows summaries, comparisons and generalizations to be made.

Interviews were conducted with 180 individuals, 78 of whom were male and 102 female. The sample was made up of lay people, dental students and dental professionals.

2.1 Sample

The study was carried out in the Midwest region of Santa Catarina, using interviews based on a semi-structured, self-explanatory questionnaire. The volunteers were divided into three groups: group 1-60 dental surgeons; group 2-60 dental academics; group 3-60 laypeople. The research subjects were of both genders, of different ages and with varying levels of education. To make up the group of academics, students from all stages of the Dentistry course at UNOESC - Joa^aba Campus were interviewed and chosen at random. For the group of professionals, questionnaires were handed out in private clinics and to teachers on the dentistry course at UNOESC - Campus de Joa^aba. Among the lay public, patients being treated at dental clinics were questioned.

The questionnaires were administered after providing information about the purpose of the study and signing the Informed Consent Form. The study was carried out after approval by the UNOESC Research Ethics Committee (No. 102.761).

For quantitative data analysis, Epi-Info software, version 07 for Windows, was used to distribute frequencies.

3. RESULTS

Among the dental professionals interviewed, 65% were male and 35% female, aged between 25 and 55, with the majority having postgraduate degrees. Of the academics, 33.9% were male and 66.1% female, with the majority (93.3%) aged up to 24. The majority of the lay people interviewed were female (71.9%) and 28% male. Of these, a large proportion (78.3%) had between 1° incomplete and 2° complete schooling.

Table 1. Socio-demographic characteristics of the sample

	Lay Populating	%	Academics	%	Professionals	%
Gender	Male	28,1%	Male	33,9%	Male	65%

	Female	71,9%	Female	66,1%	Female	35%
	1a24	20,0%	1a24	93,3%	1 a24	-
Age (years)	25a34	26,6%	25a34	5%	25a34	38,3%
	35a44	28,3%	35a44	1,67%	35a44	25,0%
	45a54	11,6%	45a54	-	45a54	35,0%
	55or more	13,3%	55or more	-	55or more	1,67%
	1st grade incomplete	25%			Graduating incomplete	100%
	1st grade completed	8,33%				
Education	High school incomplete	15%			Graduating student complete	6,6%
	Completed high school	30%				
	Graduating incomplete	13,3%			Postgraduate student	93,3%
	Graduating student complete	3,33%				
	Postgraduate	5,0%				

Source: the authors

Table 2. Percentage distribution of dental professionals' knowledge of the Human Tooth Bank.

Questions	Yes	No	Don't know/White
Are you in favor of organ donation?	100%	-	-
Would you donate organs?	89,8%	-	10,1%
Are you a donor?	63,4%	31,6%	5%
Do you know a donor?	61,7%	38,3%	-
Would I get an organ?	98,33%	-	1,67%
Do you know a receiver?	46,7%	53,3%	-
Do you know an organ or tissue bank?	63,33%	35%	1,67%
Do you think the tooth is an organ?	98,33%	1,67%	-
Do you know a tooth bank?	72,9%	27,1%	-
Do you think a tooth bank is important?	96,6%	-	3,4%
Would you donate extracted teeth to a tooth bank?	98,3%	1,7%	-
Would you use BD teeth for restorative material?	58,3%	20%	21,7%
Do you know where the teeth go?	65%	31,6%	3,4%
extracted in dental clinics?			
Did you use human teeth during your undergraduate studies?	91,6%	8,4%	-

Do you know the origin of the teeth you used?	61,1%	37,21%	1,69%

With dental professionals as the subjects of the survey, all agree with organ donation, 89.8% would donate their own organs, and 98.33% would receive organs if necessary. With regard to the dental element, 98.33% consider the tooth to be an organ of the human body and 72.9% said they were aware of the tooth bank and agreed that this institution is important for the correct disinfection and storage of extracted teeth. During graduation, 91.6% used teeth as teaching material, however only 61.1% of respondents know the origin of the teeth that were used.

Table 3. Percentage distribution of dental students' knowledge of the Human Tooth Bank.

Questions	Yes	No	Don't know/White
Are you in favor of organ donation?	98%	2%	
Would you donate organs?	84%	6%	10%
Are you a donor?	30%	58%	12%
Do you know a donor?	46%	50%	4%
Would I get an organ?	89,8%	2,04%	8,16%
Do you know a receiver?	38%	54%	8%
Do you know an organ or tissue bank?	36,8%	59,11%	4,09%
Do you think the tooth is an organ?	89,8%	6,12%	4,08%
Do you know a tooth bank?	77,55%	22,45%	
Do you think a tooth bank is important?	94%	-	6%
Would you donate extracted teeth to a tooth bank?	90%	4%	6%
Would you use BD teeth for restorative material?	52%	20%	28%
Do you know where the teeth go?	40%	52%	8%

extracted in dental clinics?			
Did you use human teeth during graduation?	86%	12%	2%
Do you know the origin of the teeth you used?	38%	62%	

Source: the authors.

With regard to academics, the questionnaire showed that the majority are in favor of organ donation (98%), 84% would donate their organs and 89.8% would be organ recipients if necessary. With regard to extracted teeth, 89.8% recognize that the dental element is an organ of the human body and would donate their teeth to a BDH after extraction; 52% would use the stored teeth as restorative material. It can be seen that 77.55% of the academics interviewed are aware of the tooth bank set up at the university, but 40% replied that they don't know the correct destination for the dental elements and root remains extracted in the dental clinics.

Table 4. Percentage distribution of the lay population's knowledge of the Bank of Human teeth.

Questions	Yes	No	Don't know/White
Are you in favor of organ donation?	90,2%	9,80%	
Would you donate organs?	80,32%	13,8%	5,88%
Are you a donor?	42%	46%	12%
Do you know a donor?	25,4%	54,9%	19,7%
Would I get an organ?	80,3%	9,80%	9,8%
Do you know a receiver?	22%	72%	6%
Do you know an organ or tissue bank?	15,7%	74,5%	9,8%

Do you think the tooth is an organ?	50,9%	29,7%	19,4%
Do you know a tooth bank?	17,6%	72,5%	9,9%
Do you think a tooth bank is important?	76%	6%	18%
Would you donate extracted teeth to a tooth bank?	82,35%	11,77%	5,88%
Would you use BD teeth for restorative material?	66%	16%	18%
Do you know where the teeth go?	11,9%	76,4%	11,7%
extracted in dental clinics?			
Did you use human teeth during graduation?	-	98,4%	1,96%
Do you know the origin of the teeth you used?	-	95,65%	4,35%

Source: the authors.

With regard to lay people, the vast majority are in favor of organ donation (90.2%), 80.32% would donate organs and 80.3% would receive organs. According to the questionnaire, only 50.9% recognize the tooth as an organ of the human body, but 82.35% would donate their teeth after extraction to be stored in a BDH, and 66% would use these stored teeth as restorative material. It's worth noting that 76% of those interviewed think a tooth bank is important, but 76.4% don't know the correct destination for their teeth after extraction.

4. DISCUSSION

With the great improvement in survival and quality of life of organ transplant patients, the indications for transplants and the number of patients seeking this therapy have grown significantly over the last two decades.[10] This information is in line with this study, as it was observed that the majority of the population interviewed, regardless of their level of education, agree with organ donation.[11] . The lay population, despite having a limited level of knowledge on the subject, showed that the majority (90.2%) are in favor of organ donation, 80.32% would donate and 80.3% would receive organs if necessary. In relation to the other two groups, the opinion on organ donation is the same, i.e. the interviewees have knowledge about donation and are in favor of it, which is in line with research where the population's opinion and knowledge about organ donation can influence the organ procurement process, demonstrating that educational programs are effective in increasing interest and improving the population's opinion about donation and, consequently, increasing organ donation.[12]

The recognition of the dental element as an organ of the human body is a factor that is little considered by the majority of dental professionals and those involved in scientific research.[1] However, the results of the study showed that 98.33% of professionals and 89.8% of academics consider the dental element to be an organ of the human body, as it performs its functions in the masticatory system. It is worth noting that in the lay population this percentage fell to 50.9%. Therefore, according to this survey, professionals' knowledge is excellent, but academics and especially laypeople need to be given more information on how to recognize that the tooth can be considered an organ.

When asked if they were aware of the existence of a Human Tooth Bank, 72.9% of professionals said they were aware of the institution; among academics, 77.55% were also aware of it, and among laypeople the percentage fell to 17.6%. These results agree with Nassif[9] , that publicizing the BDH is of fundamental importance for its growth and for the development of its functions. By spreading the word, the importance of teeth can be valued, the number of donations increased and, consequently, the number of activities carried out with teeth (such as research and pre-clinical laboratory studies) and the trade in teeth reduced.

In studies carried out at Brazilian dental schools, it was observed that this type of organ bank is rarely set up. There is therefore a need for a greater campaign to provide information to schools, so that more tooth banks can be set up. In addition, public awareness campaigns should be implemented/expanded by the colleges' outreach programs, so that tooth donation becomes continuous.[6] When asked about the importance of the DBH, 96.6% of professionals agreed that it should be set up, 94% of academics and 76% of laypeople also said it was important. Ferreira[4] explains that the Tooth Bank aims to facilitate the collection, donation and loan of teeth, taking care of their origin as well as their destination, creating ideal conditions for the use of these organs, thus reducing the risk of cross-infection arising from the incorrect handling of dental organs.

During the survey, the target audience was asked about the reuse of stored teeth. According to professionals, 58.3% would use this option; among academics 52% and among laypeople 66% agree with using teeth stored in BDH to replace or reconstruct lost structures in the oral cavity. Reusing teeth as restorative material by bonding them with resin cement (biological restoration) allows for a more aesthetic finish, a smoother surface and wear similar to that of other teeth, and there is no pain or rejection in this transplant.[2]

5. FINAL CONSIDERATIONS

Based on the results obtained, it can be concluded that organ donation is well known and accepted by the three groups of individuals surveyed. In addition, the studies showed that the vast majority of dental professionals and dental students are familiar with a human tooth bank, and that they have used human teeth during their undergraduate studies for pre-clinical procedures and research, but that the lay population has little knowledge of what a tooth bank is. Of all the people questioned, the vast majority consider the dental element to be an organ of the human body and agree on the importance of a suitable place for the correct cleaning, decontamination and storage of extracted elements, i.e. a tooth bank. This study therefore suggests that tooth banks should invest in campaigns to publicize and raise awareness, passing on information to the population and encouraging the donation of dental organs.

BIBLIOGRAPHICAL REFERENCES

1. Imparato, JCT. Banco de Dentes Humanos, l.ed. Curitiba; 2003. 35-36 p.
2. Costa, SM, et al. Human teeth in dental education: origin, use, decontamination and storage by UNIMONTES academics. Rev. ABENO. 2007;7(1):6-12.
3. Poletto, MM et al. Human tooth bank: socio-cultural profile of a group of donors. RGO. 2010;58(1):91-4
4. Ferreira, EL, Fariniuk LF, Cavali AEC, Baratto FF, Ambrósio AR. Tooth banking: Ethics and legality in teaching, research and dental treatment. RBO. 2003 Mar/Apr; 60(2):120-2.
5. Pantera, EA, Schuster GS. Sterilization of extracted human teeth. Dent Mater 1990; 11:321-3
6. Begosso MP, Imparato JCP, Duarte DA. Current status of the organization of human tooth banks in dental schools in Brazil. RPG Ver Pós- Grad. 2001;8(1):23-8
7. Brazil. Law no. 9434, of February 4, 1997. Provides for the removal of organs, tissues and parts of the human body for the purposes of transplantation and treatment and makes other provisions. Diário Oficial da Uniao, Brasilia (DF); 1997 Feb 5.
8. Brazil. Ministry of Health. Resolution no. 196, of October 16, 1996. Establishes the requirements for conducting clinical research on health products using human beings. Diário Oficial da Uniao, Brasilia (DF); 1996 Oct. 16.
9. Nassif, ACS et al. Structuring a Human Tooth Bank. *Pesqui. Odontol. Bras.* 2003;17(1):70-4. ISSN 1517-7491.
10. Coelho, JCU, Parolin MB, Baretta GAP, Pimentel SK, Freitas ACT, Colman D. Donor quality of life after inter-vivos liver transplantation. Arq Gastroenterol. 2005;42:83-8.
11. Moraes, MW, Gallani MCBJ, Meneghin P. Beliefs that influence adolescents in organ donation. Rev

Esc Enferm USP. 2006;40:484-92.

12. Piccoli GB, Soragna G, Putaggio S, Mezza E, Burdese M, Vespertino E, et al. Efficacy of an educational program for secondary school students on opinions on renal transplantation and organ donation: a randomized controlled trial. Nephrol Dial Transplant. 2006;21:499-50.

ARTICLE 3:

EVALUATING THE KNOWLEDGE OF DENTAL SURGEONS WORKING IN THE MIDWEST REGION OF SANTA CATARINA ABOUT THE EXISTENCE OF THE UNOESC HUMAN TOOTH BANK

SLONGO, Isadora Lahyz[§] DALLANORA, Léa Maria Franceschi[**]

DALLANORA, Fábio José[2]

SUMMARY

The Human Tooth Bank (HDB) is a non-profit institution that must be linked to an educational institution and one of its aims is to meet academic, teaching and research needs. It is assumed that between 700 and 900 dental units are used during the course of the Dentistry course, which are used in subjects such as Anatomy, Dentistry, Endodontics and Prosthetics. The aim of this study is to measure the knowledge of dentists in the Midwest region of Santa Catarina on the subject of 'human tooth banks'. It also aims to inform the community of dentists about the existence and operation of the human tooth's bank at the University of Western Santa Catarina and to encourage the donation of dental elements. The study adopts a predominantly quantitative research approach, using a questionnaire with pre-defined questions. The sample included 100 dentists working in the Midwest region of Santa Catarina. It was observed that most dentists consider the tooth to be an organ, with 99% stating that they would donate extracted teeth to the tooth bank, but only 65% say they know of a human tooth bank and are also willing to donate extracted elements, justifying the need for a publicity campaign. Also, with regard to handling teeth, 97% of dentists have used human teeth during their undergraduate studies. The implementation of a tooth bank in universities fulfills an important ethical, moral and didactic function, storing teeth in accordance with biosafety standards, eliminating illegal trade and favoring the field of research. The DBH is the best way to comply with legislation, given the importance of using human biological material for the development of health sciences.

Keywords: Tooth. Bioethics. Human tooth bank.

1INTRODUCÁ!)

According to Pereira (2012), the creation of Human Tooth Banks (HDB) in higher education institutions in Brazil began around 2000, with the aim of minimizing the illegal trade in dental structures, as well as developing the perception of students and professionals in the field of Dentistry about Biosafety, legal issues and discussions on Bioethics. Currently, Human Tooth Banks are regulated by the National Research Ethics Council through CNS Resolution No. 441 of May 12, 2011.

Biological material repositories or banks are collections where human cells, tissues, organs or physiological fluids are kept and stored to meet surgical, teaching or research needs (MOTTA-MURGUIA; SARUWATARI-ZAVALA, 2016).

Imparato (2003) and Motta-Murguia and Saruwatari-Zavala (2016), emphasize that the BDH is a non-profit institution, which must be linked to a college, university or other institution. Its purpose is to meet academic needs by providing human teeth for research or teaching activities. The storage period for human biological material in a Biobank is indefinite, and the maintenance of its accreditation is subject to compliance with current regulations (BRASIL, 2011).

Imparato (2003) mentions that, in fact, the tooth is an organ of the human body and, as such, is subject to the Brazilian Transplant Law (Law 9434 of 04/02/1997), which provides for a penalty of 3 to 8 years in prison and a fine for anyone who removes, post-mortem, organs, tissues and parts of the human body of an unidentified person. The Penal Code also provides for a penalty of 1 to 3 years in prison for those who violate a grave (Article 210) and the National Health Council requires the free and informed consent of the subjects as a form of "respect for human dignity" (Resolution 196 of 10/10/1996), CNS Resolution 441 of May 12, 2011 reinforces the need for the Free and Informed Consent form.

According to Zanatta et al. (2014), Unoesc's Human Tooth Bank was structured in accordance with Research Project No. 1149/09, Process No. 1255/10 and Resolution No. 01/CG/11, respecting the institution's statutes. It has its own internal regulations and a physical space duly equipped for disinfecting and storing dental elements, in accordance with university policy. In order for the BDH to operate perfectly, it has a

---

[§] Dentistry student at the Universidade do Oeste de Santa Catarina.

[**] Professor of Dentistry at the Universidade do Oeste de Santa Catarina.

protocol for receiving donations, requesting and using permanent and deciduous human teeth.

When teaching dentistry, the use of human teeth is essential for learning. Calculating mathematically, in the Dentistry course at UNOESC .loacaba a class of 30 students per semester needs an average of 700 to 900 units for teaching throughout the course, in components such as Anatomy, Dentistry, Endodontics, Prosthesis, among others. Skelton-Macedo et al. (2014) mention that many elements have been employed so that students can have contact with their future field of work, and this means feeding each of the more than 200 undergraduate dentistry courses in the country. All the teeth used in the dentistry course must come from a tooth bank, as they are human organs and subject to the guidelines of the organ donation law. The BDH follows these guidelines and the teeth are properly cleaned and stored.

The aim of this study was to measure awareness of the existence of the BDH and, at the same time, to inform the community of dentists about the existence and functioning of the human tooth bank at the University of Western Santa Catarina, because tooth collection is not widely disseminated among dentists.

2 MATERIALS AND METHODS

The study in question adopts a predominantly quantitative research perspective, as it uses standardized data that allows summaries, comparisons and generalizations to be drawn up.

The study was approved under protocol 1.380.568 by the Research Ethics Committee of Unoesc HUST (CEP). The sample consisted of dentists working in the Midwest region of Santa Catarina, chosen at random. The participants answered a questionnaire consisting of 13 closed questions, adapted from the questionnaire used in (PINTO, 2009), and 2 open questions (age and time since graduation), which deals with organ donation and the recognition of teeth as human organs, and the correct destination of extracted teeth. The questionnaire was administered in person in March 2016.

After administering the questionnaire, *a flyer* (Image 1) was handed out containing information about the UNOESC Human Tooth Bank and a donation form, along with an appropriate container for the possible collection of dental elements.

A total of 128 dentists were randomly selected, duly registered with the Regional Dental Council, with the inclusion criterion being their residence in the Midwest of Santa Catarina, and the exclusion criterion being all those who did not agree to the free and informed consent form, 28 of whom did not agree to sign it. The sample included 100 volunteer dentists of both genders, aged between 21 and 66.

The data obtained from the survey was organized into tables and treated statistically using the chi-square and *Kruskal-Wallis* tests.

Image 1 - Promotional *flyer*

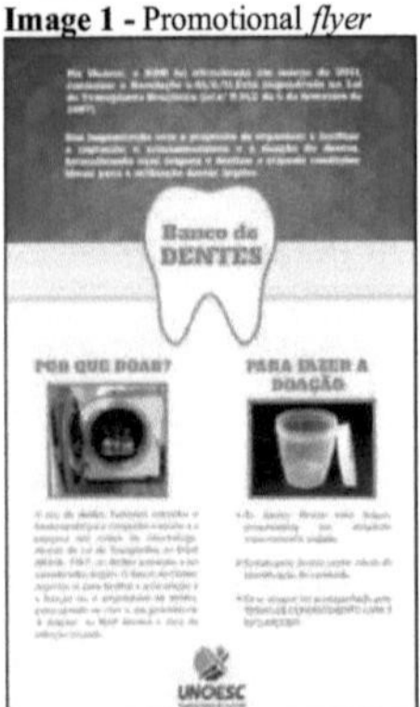

Source: the authors.

3 RESULTS

The participation of dental surgeons resulted in 100 completed questionnaires. Of those interviewed, 43% were male and 57% were female, with 51% of the sample having been trained for more than 10 years. The answers to the closed questions in the questionnaire are shown in Table 1.

Table 1. Percentage distribution of the knowledge of dentists in the Midwest of Santa Catarina about the Human Tooth Bank.

Questions	Yes (%)	No (%)	I didn't know

			(%)
In favor of organ donation	98	1	1
Donate organs	94	2	4
He's a donor	68	28	4
Meet a donor	70	27	3
It would receive an organ	91	4	5
You know a receiver	44	51	5
Do you know an organ or tissue bank?	47	52	1
Do you know a tooth bank	65	35	-
Used human teeth during graduation	97	3	-
Consider that the tooth is an organ	98	2	-
Do you think a tooth bank is important?	98	2	-
I would donate extracted teeth to a tooth bank	99	1	-
I would donate extracted teeth to a tooth bank	93	4	3

Source: The authors.

With regard to handling teeth, 97% of the dentists had used human teeth during their degree and 3% had not. Regarding the donation of teeth, 99% would donate them to the tooth bank.

With regard to being in favor of donating teeth, 98 of those who said they were in favor of organ donation, 97 said they would donate extracted teeth to the tooth bank and only 1 said he would not donate extracted teeth to the tooth bank. One (1) interviewee also said that he did not consider a tooth bank to be important, but stated that he would donate extracted teeth to the tooth bank, as can be seen in TABLE 2.

Table 2- Distribution of the association between "considers a tooth bank important" *versus* "would donate extracted teeth to a tooth bank".

		Do you know a tooth bank		
		Yes	No	p*
Do you think a tooth bank is important?	Yes	98	0	
	No	1	1	<0,001
*Chi-squared				

Of the 98 interviewees who claimed to be in favor of organ donation, only 92 said they would donate their own teeth to the BDH, 3 would not, and 3 said they didn't know. There is a statistically significant difference, as shown in Table 3.

Table 3- Distribution of the association between Is in favor of organ donation *versus* Would donate a tooth to the BDH".

		Yes	I would donate a tooth for BDH		
			No	You don't know	p*
Are you in favor of	Yes	92	3	3	
donated from	No	0	1	0	<0,001
organs	You don't know	1	0	0	
*Kruskal-wallis					

In the bivariate analyses between knowledge of an organ or tissue bank and knowledge of a tooth bank, the results were statistically significant (Table 4).

Table 4 - Distribution of the association between knowledge of an organ or tissue bank and knowledge of a tooth bank.

		Do you know a tooth bank		
		Yes	No	p*
	Yes	38	9	
Do you know an organ or tissue bank?	No	26	26	0,004
	You don't know	1	0	
*Kruskal-wallis				

Table 5 shows that there is no statistically significant difference between the individuals who would donate extracted teeth and those who know of a human tooth bank, and this is a positive finding, since the 47 who said they knew of an organ and tissue bank would also donate extracted teeth to the tooth bank.

Table 5 - Distribution of the association between knowledge of an organ or tissue bank and willingness to donate extracted teeth to a tooth bank

		I would donate extracted teeth to a tooth bank		p*
		Yes	No	
	Yes	47	0	
Do you know an organ or tissue bank?	No	51	1	0,932
	You don't know	1	0	
*Kruskal-Wallis				

There was no statistically significant correlation between time since graduation and age group and the questions about being in favor of organ donation and knowing a tooth bank.

The average age and average time since graduation were higher among those who said they knew of an organ or tissue bank.

Table 6 shows the bivariate analysis between the questions "Are you in favor of organ donation?" and "Would you donate organs?" The result was statistically significant and $p < 0.001$. Three people who answered "I don't know" to the question "Would you donate organs?" claimed to be in favor of organ donation.

Table 6 - Distribution of the association between the questions "Would you donate organs" and "Are you in favor of organ donation"

		In favor of organ donation			
		Yes	No	You don't know	P
	Yes	94	0	0	
Donate organs	No	1	1	0	**0,001**
	You don't know	3	0	1	
*Kruskal-Wallis					

During the period of this study, only 68 dental elements were collected for the UNOESC Human Tooth Bank, with the DCs verbally telling the interviewer that they had already donated or disposed of the extracted dental elements in contaminated waste.

4 DISCUSSION

Costa et al. (2007) mention that in 1997, with the formulation of the Transplant Law in Brazil, teeth were recognized as organs. In fact, the tooth is an organ of the human body and, as such, is subject to the Brazilian Transplant Law (law 9434 of 04/02/1997) (NASSIF et al, 2003). In order to strengthen the transplant law, the Ministry of Health regulated Ordinance 904/00, which creates banks of human osteo-fascio-chondroligamentous tissues for therapeutic or scientific purposes (BRASIL, 2000).

In this study, 98% of those interviewed said they were in favor of organ donation. Of these, only 92% said that they would donate a tooth of their own to a human tooth bank, 3% said that they would not donate and 3% that they did not know; these data were statistically significant. These data corroborate a previous study by (PINTO et al., 2009), in which 94% of dental professionals said they were in favor of organ donation, but only 90% would donate their own teeth to a human tooth bank. This is an intriguing fact, as 98% of those interviewed consider the human tooth to be an organ.

Pinto et al. (2009) point out that, following this law on the valorization of teeth, some aspects "concern the dental pulp, which will also be studied for possible stem cell donors, along with cells from the brain, eyes, skin and muscles". The valorization of the tooth as an organ aims to comply with the law that "regulates the removal of organs, tissues and parts of the human body for the purposes of transplantation, treatment and other procedures". (BRASIL, 1997)

According to Pereira (2012), the creation of Human Tooth Banks in Higher Education Institutions in Brazil began around the year 2000, with the aim of minimizing the illegal trade in dental structures, as well as developing the perception of students and professionals in the field of Dentistry about Biosafety, legal issues and discussions on Bioethics. According to Zanatta et al. (2014), the BDH at UNOESC was implemented in 2011, and only 65% of those interviewed were aware of the institution.

In a study carried out by Marodin, França and Tannous (2012), it was found that 70.6% of students at universities in Rio de Janeiro and 46.9% of students in Sao Paulo had bought teeth for their academic activities in 2001. Also in the same study, the results indicate that most orders for teeth were placed in cemeteries through gravediggers, indicating that this "crime" is constantly being committed. This study shows that 99% of those interviewed are willing to donate extracted teeth, thus contributing to the expansion of the Human Teeth Bank and reducing illegal trade. The New Code of Dental Ethics, approved by the
CFO Resolution 118/2012 prohibits, in its Chap. XIII art. 35, "participating directly or indirectly in the commercialization of human organs and tissues", and in Chap. XIV on the donation, transplantation and banking of organs, tissues and biomaterials. (BRASIL, 2012)

According to Nassif et al. (2003), the purpose of the Human Tooth Bank is to meet academic needs by providing human teeth for research and teaching activities. In a study carried out by Freitas et al. (2010), of the 33 journals that made up the final sample, 14 published articles whose methodologies reported the use of extracted teeth, totaling 254 articles and 11,841 teeth. In this study, 97% of dental surgeons used human teeth during their undergraduate studies. Pereira (2012) points out that the use of dental units in undergraduate courses is a necessity and a reality in both dental teaching and dental research. UNOESC's Human Tooth Bank has a collection of approximately 12,000 units of dental elements, available for students to use in teaching practice, teaching and research.

The creation of Human Tooth Banks in Brazilian Dental Teaching Institutions should be the best way to comply with current legislation on research involving human beings (BRASIL, 1996), considering the importance of using human biological material for the development of health sciences (BRASIL, 2011). Most of the DCs interviewed (99%) considered a DBH to be important, agreeing with Marin (2005), who emphasizes that its relevance is unquestionable and that only a regularly structured DBH can provide for the safe use and storage of teeth intended for student activities, teachers or interested dental surgeons.

Zucco et al. (2006) state that there is a great deal of resistance on the part of professionals to donating their private collections of teeth, which is probably due to a lack of knowledge about how the Human Tooth Bank works or even exists. However, when asked about donating dental elements, 93% of dentists in the Midwest of Santa Catarina would donate their own teeth and 98% said that they would donate elements extracted in their clinics to the BDH, which is the vast majority, which is also in line with the study by Pinto et al. (2009). In this study, 65% of the interviewees reported knowing about a Human Tooth Bank, representing just over half of the interviewees, in contrast to Pinto et al. (2009), where only 28% of the DCs interviewed reported knowing about a HDB. However, during the interviews, only 63 dental elements were found with the appropriate terms of donation, which is a low percentage. This shows that there is a lack of information about the existence and importance of HDFs, making it important to publicize them.

In dentistry courses and postgraduate programs, extracted dental elements are constantly used by students and professors for pre-clinical training and the development of scientific research. Considering that 97 dental surgeons had used human teeth during their undergraduate studies, but that only 65% said they knew of a human tooth bank, this study is in line with Silva et al. (2001), who stated that teeth of unknown origin are used indiscriminately and that they are often not decontaminated in any way, and both are in line with what was observed by Pinto et al. (2009), where 90% of professionals and 86% of undergraduates reported having used extracted human teeth during their dental studies; on the other hand, in their study, 72% of dental surgeons and 98% of undergraduates were unaware of the existence of a BDH. This finding is very worrying because of the risk of cross-infection when handling this material, whose storage and disinfection methods are unknown.

Gomes et al. (2013) state that dental organ reassembly is still a common occurrence in dental care establishments and, most of the time, there is still no appropriate destination for this extracted element. According to González-Pita et al. (2014), the protocols that guarantee the functioning of the BDH eliminate unhealthy practices, adopt biosafety practices and make it possible to standardize and reproduce the procedures for each sample, in addition to keeping the tissues in better condition. In this study, the number of interviewees who thought the BDH was important and would donate extracted teeth to the BDH was significant, which shows that the BDH is achieving its objectives of disseminating and collecting teeth for teaching and research through its operational procedures.

According to Vanzelli, Ramos and Imparato (2003), the ethical and legal way of using human teeth, whether in research, clinical or laboratory procedures, needs to be in the mindset of all academics, teachers and researchers in the field of dentistry, for the rational use of extracted teeth. Human tooth banks are proving to be an ethical way of controlling the use of extracted human teeth.

5 CONCLUSION

The implementation of human tooth banks in universities fulfills an important ethical, moral and didactic function, storing teeth in accordance with biosafety standards. It was observed that most dentists in the Midwest of Santa Catarina consider teeth to be organs and are also willing to donate extracted elements to the Human Tooth Bank. However, knowledge of the existence of a Biobank in the UNOESC by individuals from this segment is small, and it is pertinent to carry out publicity campaigns.

ABSTRACT

The Biobank ofhuman teeth repositorie of Unoesc is a non-profit organization that has as one of its purposes to fulfill academic requirements, Teaching and Research. It is assumed that in the Dentistry course are used 700-900 dental units, which are used in curriculum components such as Anatomy, Dentistry, Endodontics and Prosthodontics. This study aims to measure the knowledge of Dental Surgeons of Middle Western region of Santa Catarina on the theme 'biobank of human teeth', also aims to disseminate in experience dentists the existence and functioning of the Biobank of human teeth repositorie at University ofWest of Santa Catarina and encourage the donation of teeth. The study mainly adopts the perspective of quantitative research, adopting a questionnaire with pre-defined questions. The sample included the participation of 100 Dentists working in the Midwest of Santa Catarina, and 99% say they would donate extracted teeth to the bank of teeth, but only 65% say they know a Biobank of human teeth, justifying the need of publicity campaigns. The Biobank is the best way to comply with the law, and fulfills an important ethical, moral and didactic function, storing the teeth according to the bio-security standards, eliminating illegal trade, and encouraging the field of research, that considering the importance of use ofhuman biological material for the development of life sciences.

Keywords: Tooth. Bioethics. Biobank of human teeth.

REFERENCES

BRAZIL, **CFO - Federal Code of Dentistry**, 2012. 20p. Available at: <http://cfo.org.br/wp-content/uploads/2009/09/codigo_etica.pdf>. Accessed on: April 21, 2016.

BRASIL. Portaria nº 904/00, Ministério da Saúde de16de agosto de 2000. **Diário Oficial da União**, Brasilia (DF); 2000. Available at: <www.conselho.saude. gov.br>. Accessed on: May 1, 2016.

BRASIL. Resoluçao n. 196, de16de outubro de 1996. **Diário Oficial da União**, Brasilia, DF, October 16, 1996. Available at: <www.conselho.saude.gov.br>. Accessed on: 03 May 2016.

BRAZIL. Resolution no. 441, of May 12, 2011. **Diário Oficial da União**, Brasilia, DF, May 12, 2011. Available at: <www.conselho.saude.gov.br>. Accessed on: May 3, 2016.

BRAZIL. Resolution tf 9.434, of February 4, 1997. **Organ Transplant Law**. Brasilia (DF), May 12, 2011. Available at: <http://www.iusbrasil.com.br/topicos/11454097/artigo-4-da-lei-n-9434-de-04-de-fevereiro- de-1997>. Accessed on: April 29, 2016.

COSTA, S. de M. et al. Human teeth in dental education: origin, use, decontamination and storage / by UNIMONTES academics. **Revista da Abeno,** Londrina, v. 7, n. 1, p.6-12,jan. 2007. Quarterly.

FREITAS, A. B. D. A. de. Use of extracted teeth in dental research published in Brazilian journals with free online access: a study from the perspective of bioethics. **Arquivos em Odontologia,** Belo Horizonte, v.46, n.3, p. 136-143, jul. 2010.

GOMES, GM. Use of human teeth: ethical and legal aspects. Rev Gaúcha Odontol., Porto Alegre, v.61, p. 477-483,jul./dez., 2013

GONZÁLEZ-PITA, L. C. et al. Protocols designed for the tooth biobank of the National University of Colombia. **Acta Odontológica Colombiana,** Bogotá, v. 2, n. 4, p.79-93, jul. 2014.

IMPARATO, J. C. P. **Banco de Dentes Humanos**. Curitiba: Editora Maio, 2003. p. 35-36.

SKELTON-MACEDO, M. C. Teleodontology in the process of dissemination and implementation of Human Tooth Banks. **Revista da Abeno,** Londrina, v.14, n.1, p.30-37,jan. 2014. Quarterly.

MACHADO, M. R.; GARRIDO, R. G. Teeth as Source of Stem Cells: an Alternative to Ethical Dilemmas. **Revista de Bioética y Derecho.** Barcelona, v. 31,n. 1, p.66-80, May 2014.

MARIN, E. A. et al. Structuring the Bank of Deciduous Human Teeth at the Federal University of Santa Maria / RS / Brazil. **Revista da Faculdade de Odontologia8,** Passo Fundo, v. 10, n. 2, p.7-9, jul. 2005.

MARODIN, G.; FRANÇA, P. H. C.; TANNOUS, G. S. A Resoluçao do Conselho Nacional de Saúde n.196/96. In: REGO, Sergio; PALÁCIOS, Marisa. **Research ethics committees: theory and practice.** Rio de Janeiro: National School of Public Health (ensp/fiocruz), 2012. p. 121-137.

MOREIRA, L. et al. Human Tooth Bank for Teaching and Research in Odontology. **Rev. Fac. Odontol. Porto Alegre,** Porto Alegre, v. 50, n. 1, p.34-37,jan. 2009.

MOTTA-MURGUIA, L.; SARUWATARI-ZAVALA, G. Mexican Regulation of Biobanks. **The Journal Of Law, Medicine & Ethics,** Boston, v. 44, n. 1, p. 58-67, Mar. 2016.

NASSIF, A. C. da S. et al. Structuring a Human Tooth Bank. **Pesqui Odontol Bras,** São Paulo, v. 17, p.70-74, 2003.

PEREIRA, D. Q. Banco de Dentes Humanos no Brasil: revisão de literatura. **Revista da Abeno,** Londrina, v.12, n.2, p.178-184,jul. 2012.

PEREIRA, D. Q. **Survey of tooth banks in dentistry courses in Brazil and experience in creating a human tooth bank at the State University of Feira de Santana - Bahia.** 2012. 110f Thesis (Doctorate) - Medicine Course, Bahia Medical School, Salvador, 2012.

PINTO, L. et al. Popular, Academic and Professional Knowledge about the Human Tooth Bank. **Pesquisa Brasileira em Odontopediatria e Clínica Integrada,** Paraiba, v. 9,n. 1, p.101-106,jan. 2009. Available at: < Available at: http://www.redalyc.org/articulo.oa7idM3712848016>. Accessed on: 14nov. 2015.

SILVA, A. C. da C. et al. Quantitative survey of human teeth requested in the first semester of 2001 in dentistry courses in the state of Pernambuco. **An Fac Odontol Univ Fed Pernamb,** Pernambuco, v. 11, n. 1, p.29-32,jan. 2001.

TELLES, P. D. et al. Pulp tissue from primary teeth: new source of stem cells. **J Appl Oral Sci,** Bauru, v. 19, n.3, p.189-194, 2011.

VANZELLI, M.; RAMOS, D. L. de P.; IMPARATO, J. C. P. Valuing the tooth as an organ. In: IMPARATO, José Carlos Pettorossi. **Human tooth bank.** Curitiba: Editora Maio, 2003. p. 33-37.

ZANATTA, C. et al. Implementation of the human teeth bank (BDH) of the dentistry course at the University of Western Santa Catarina. **Unoesc & Ciencia [online],** Joaçaba, v. 5, n.1, jul. 2014.

ZUCCO, D. et al. Evaluation of the level of knowledge of UNIVILLE Dentistry undergraduates about the use of extracted teeth and the tooth bank. **Revista Sul Brasileira de Odontologia,** Joinville, v. 3, n. 1, p.54-58, jul. 2006.

Article 4

INFLUENCE OF DIFFERENT STORAGE SOLUTIONS ON THE BOND STRENGTH OF AN ADHESIVE SYSTEM AND COMPOSITE RESIN TO DENTAL ENAMEL

Georgia Cesca*

Lea Maria F. Dallanora* *

Leonardo Flores Luthi***

SUMMARY

This study evaluated the difference between storing human teeth in distilled water and in a solution of distilled water plus preservative, which in this study was methylparaben, in its commercial form as Nipagim®. The study used 30 human third molars from the tooth bank at the University of Western Santa Catarina - Joacaba Campus. The physical properties of the dental elements, stored in distilled water and distilled water plus the preservative methylparaben, were observed with regard to microtraction based on the adhesion of the Single Bond adhesive system to the enamel between the substrate and the composite resin. The Tukey statistical test showed that there was no difference between groups Gl, G2 and G3, thus concluding that the

preservative methylparaben does not interfere with the adhesion between composite resin and dental enamel.
Keywords: Microtracking. Methylparaben. Tooth bank. Composite resin.

1 INTRODUCTION

Teeth, like other human organs, have a specific function in the human body and are made up of different types of tissue (JUNQUEIRA E CARNEIRO, 1999). Once extracted, they can be used in scientific research and treatments, thus adding to the evolution in the view of the tooth as an integral organ of the human body (BEGOSSO; IMPARATO; DUARTE, 2001).

Always linked to an educational institution, the human tooth bank (HDB) plays an important role in terms of research and studies at a dental university, as it is legalized and provides good storage conditions for human teeth. With this, the BDH complies with the requirements of the Research Ethics Committee, which does not approve research using human teeth whose origin is not proven or legalized (NASSIF, 2003).

In order to store human teeth in a tooth bank, they need to be sterilized correctly and stored properly; however, the literature is divergent and confusing when it comes to sterilizing and disinfecting teeth. The most common types of storage are: serum, dry, under refrigeration and under refrigeration in water, given that some types of solution used can interfere with the chemical and physical characteristics of tooth structures (BEGOSSO; IMPARATO; DUARTE, 2001).

The preparation, sealing and methods of disinfecting and sterilizing teeth can vary according to the research and, above all, the purpose for which the teeth are intended. Another important aspect is the fact that freshly extracted teeth are considered a potential source of cross-infection and contamination and should therefore be stored in conditions that allow them to maintain their physical properties and be properly decontaminated before being used in laboratory research activities (Silva et al., 2006). It is also up to the BDH to ensure that cross-infection is eliminated when these dental elements are handled incorrectly (MIRANDA; BUENO, 2012).

Knowing that there are various methods of decontaminating and storing teeth, the use of these agents should not modify important characteristics of dental tissue, such as dentin bond strength and microfiltering (Moreira et al., 2009). In dentin, the influence of disinfection methods seems to be different than in enamel, since there is a greater organic content represented mainly by collagen fibers (Haller et al., 1993).

The use of dental elements in in vitro laboratory studies contributes to the development of new dental techniques and materials (FARAH et al., 2010; MANTON et al., 2010). Although these studies have improved understanding of the demineralizing and remineralizing process, the complex nature of the oral cavity cannot be simulated (SRINIVASAN et al, 2010). For this reason, in dentistry, the search for laboratory situations that simulate the conditions of the oral environment is an important factor in the correct development of research. Maintaining the normal condition of this substrate is essential in order to achieve the closest possible reproduction of the situations that occur in the oral cavity (Silva et al., 2006).

There is no standard storage medium to be used for preserving teeth after extraction. For this reason, studies using similar materials on the same type of substrate and showing different results are likely to occur due to the influence of other variables, such as the type of disinfectant used, storage, time and type of substance used to store the tooth (Silva et al., 2006). Thus, there is a clear need for standardization when it comes to storing teeth in tooth banks, but it is difficult to obtain a solution that meets the needs without altering the properties of the dental organ (CAMPREGHER, 2007).

Methylparaben is a paraben that is effective over a wide pH range (4-8) and has great antimicrobial action. It is presented as a crystalline, almost odorless and tasteless powder that is used as a preservative in food, cosmetic and pharmaceutical formulations. Therefore, in this study, the aim is to use it as a method of dental storage, a solution prepared with distilled water and methylparaben (Nipagim®) (GIL; BRANDÁO, 2007).

Composite resin is currently the most widely used material for direct esthetic restorations (Michelon et al., 2009). The development of techniques and materials that facilitate this restorative procedure has contributed to the popularization of aesthetic restorations with composite resin (Vieira et al., 2002). After acid etching, adhesive practice on enamel provides bonding to the restorative resin through the mechanism of micromechanical embrittlement. The clinical success of this bond is related to the enamel's inorganic composition of 86% and the formation of extensions of the adhesive resin, called tags (Nakabayashi et al., 1992).

In this study, dental elements were evaluated with regard to the micro-translation test on the bond strength between enamel and composite resin in teeth stored in two different solutions and a comparison was made, to see if there is a difference between storing human teeth in distilled H2O (group G1) and in distilled H2O plus the preservative methylparaben (groups G2 and G3) in terms of resin adhesion to tooth enamel in microtreatment tests over a period of 1 day and 30 days. In this context, the importance of this research arises, in order to prove whether or not methylparaben can alter the adhesion of the resin to the substrate, as seen through the microtranion test.

2 MATERIAL AND METHOD

This is an analytical study with a quantitative approach and experimental research in the laboratory (in vitro study). It was carried out in the tooth bank of the University of Western Santa Catarina in Joanaba (storage), and in the research laboratory of the pre-clinic II - Dentistry (micro-transplant test).

The research was carried out using a sample of 30 healthy third molars (BDH UNOESC - Joanaba), stored in glass jars with lids in distilled water (UNOESC Distiller - Joacaba campus) and in 0.2% Methylparaben Solution (NIPAGIM®) under refrigeration.

The 30 dental elements from the BDH complied with the biosafety storage standards suggested by Imparato (2003). The sample was divided into 3 groups: Gl, G2 and G3. Group Gl consisted of 10 teeth stored in distilled water; group G2, 10 teeth stored in distilled H2O plus methylparaben for 1 day and group G3, 10 teeth stored in distilled H2O plus methylparaben for 30 days.

After this, resin restorations were made on all the teeth without differentiating between groups. Firstly, the enamel was roughened and then the restoration was made with Opallis A2 enamel composite resin (FGM - Joinville - Santa Catarina), treated with 37% phosphoric acid for 30 seconds, washed and dried for the same time. A layer of Single Bond adhesive (3M - Sumaré - Sao Paulo), applied with a microbrush, air jet from a distance until the solvent evaporated, another layer of adhesive, air jet and 10-second polymerization of the adhesive (Gnatus Optilight Plus light-curing device). Finally, each resin increment was light-cured for 30 seconds and then over-cured for 40 seconds.

The tooth/resin set was cut on the Labcut 1010 (ODEME equipamentos médicos e odontológicos - Joacaba, Santa Catarina, Brazil) serial cutting machine under constant cooling with water, thus obtaining specimens measuring 1 mm wide x 1 mm high and approximately 0.5 cm long, which were used for the microtensile tests.

The EMIC universal mechanical testing machine (EMIC - Sao Jose do Pinhais - Paraná, Brazil) was used to carry out the microtensile test. The specimens were positioned in the device with the aid of cyanocrylate-based glue (Super Bonder Gel, Loctite Ltda., Piracicaba, SP, Brazil). A traction speed of 0.5 mm/min was used until rupture with a 100N load cell. The specimens were taken to total rupture, thus obtaining the microtensile strength values in MPa.

After the results were obtained and tabulated, they were submitted to the ANOVA and Tukey statistical tests at a 5% significance level.

3 RESULTS

Given the research carried out, it was possible to observe the average values using the Tukey statistical test (Table 1), thus finding a statistical difference between the following groups: G2 and G3 p=0.023.

When comparing group G1 with group G2, no statistical difference was found p= 0.168. Also, between group G1 and group G3, no statistical difference was found p= 0.820.

Table: Shows average values and standard deviation for Stress in (Mpa).

Group	Average voltage values
Gl- Distilled water	36.22 (± ll.97)AB
G2 - Nipagin l dia	46.25(± 12.50) AD
G3 - Nipagin 30 days	32.04(± l4.89)BC

Different letters show statistical differences according to Tukey's test P<0.05%.

Table 2 shows the percentage values of the type of fracture that occurred when the specimens were broken in the microtensile test. Group G1 showed 76.92% fracture in the adhesive/enamel region and 23.03% fracture in the bond line. Group G2 showed 91.6% fracture in the adhesive/enamel region and 8.33% fracture in the bond line, while group G3 showed 50% fracture in each type.

Table 2: Percentage values of the type of fracture found when the specimens were broken in the microtensile tests.

Group	Adhesive/enamel	Union Line
Gl - Distilled water	76,92%	23,07%
G2 - Nipagin 1 dia	91,6%	8,33%
G3 - Nipagin 30 days	50%	50%

4 DISCUSSION

This study evaluated the influence of two different storage solutions on the bond strength of an adhesive system and composite resin to the enamel of human teeth stored in distilled H_2O and 0.2% methylparaben solution. The teeth were cleaned, decontaminated and sterile, in accordance with current literature (IMPARATO, 2003).

All the elements of the study were sterilized in an autoclave at 130°C for homogeneity. This agrees with the study by Silva et al. (2006), who concluded that the use of an autoclave seems to be the most reliable method for disinfecting teeth and has no influence on the adhesive strength of teeth.

According to the results of this study, we can see that group G1 stored in distilled H_2O and groups G2 and G3 stored in methylparaben solution also showed a good pattern of resin adhesion strength to enamel, as there was no statistical difference between group G1 compared to groups G2 and G3 (Table 1). Goddis et al. (1993) reported the need to keep these organs in a humid environment so as not to dehydrate their structures, so one of the options is to store them in a distilled water solution, even though research indicates an increase in dentin permeability, there was no influence on the strength of adhesion to enamel.

In the present study, we found that the difference between group G1 (distilled H_2O) and group G2, where the teeth were stored for 1 day in methylparaben solution, did not vary statistically with p= 0.168, and between group G1 and G3 there was no significant variation as the index was p=0.820, but when we compared group G2 (stored for 1 day) with group G3 (stored for 30 days) there was a statistical value of p=0.023,023, which agrees with the study by Silva (2006) who compared several authors on the influence of the storage substance on the adhesion of restorative materials to the dental substrate, where most of the studies showed an influence of the storage period of the teeth on the adhesion values of the restorative material to the tooth. In conclusion, the solutions used to store human teeth in tooth banks influence the changes that may occur in the dental substrate.

According to Ghersel (2001), the storage medium used for human teeth can cause alterations to the tooth surface, which can be chemical and optical and affect adhesive strength. In this study, the tests carried out showed that the storage medium used was effective in not altering adhesion, since there was no significant difference in adhesion to tooth enamel between groups G1 and G2 p= 0.168, G1 and G3 p= 0.820, as shown in Table 1.

Among the substances normally used for storage, distilled water, thymol in different concentrations and physiological solution have not been shown to influence adhesive strength (Aquilino *et al.* 1987, Williams and Svare 1995, Silva etal., 2006). Dallanora et al. (2012) in their study found no statistical difference in microhardness when comparing the distilled water group (A1) and the 0.2% methylparaben solution group (A2) p=0.064, regardless of the number of months the teeth were stored in the different solutions, which supports further research with methylparaben, This study showed that distilled water and the solution of distilled water plus methylparaben presented a statistical index between groups G1 and G3 p= 0.820, which is not statistically significant, demonstrating that the solution does not interfere with enamel adhesion.

The non-interference of methylparaben in adhesive strength was also proven in this study, where the average tension values were 36.22 (± 11.97) in group G1, 46.25 (± 12.50) in group G2 and 32.04 (± 14.89) in group G3. The comparison between the groups was not statistically significant.

Pupo et al. (2010), comparing some authors, states that the microtensile test is chosen because it allows for a better distribution of tension at the adhesive interface, when compared to conventional shear or tensile tests, reducing the number of cohesive fractures in the substrate, we observed that as shown in Table 2, Group G1 showed 76.92% fracture between enamel/adhesive and 23.03% fracture at the bond line, while Group G2 showed 91.6% fracture between enamel/adhesive and 8.33% fracture at the bond line and Group G3 showed 50% in each type of fracture, which agrees with the studies presented.

5 CONCLUSION

The 0.2% methylparaben solution proved to be effective as a storage solution for dental elements, as it did not interfere with the adhesion of the composite resin to the enamel. However, it is suggested that further research be carried out evaluating the adhesion index to the dentin substrate and with groups of teeth stored for longer (90 and 120 days).

INFLUENCE OF DIFFERENT STORAGE SOLUTIONS IN UNION RESISTANCE OF A COMPOSITE RESIN SYSTEM AND ROUND THE DENTAL ENAMEL

ABSTRACT

The present study evaluated the difference in storage of human teeth in distilled water and in a solution of distilled water plus a preservative, which in this study was Methylparaben, commercial form which presents itself as nipagim ®. Thus, for the development of the research were used 30/3 molars teeth bank, installed at the Universidade do Oeste de Santa Catarina - Campus Joaçaba. We observed the physical properties of dental elements stored in distilled water and distilled water plus the preservative methylparaben in relation to microtensile based on the adhesiveness to enamel system adevivo Single Bond between substrate and composite resin. Before the survey, it was observed by the Tukey statistical test, there is no difference between the groups G1, G2 and G3, thereby concluding that the preservative methylparaben does not interfere with adhesion between composite resin and enamel.

Keywords: Microtensile. Methylparaben. Bank of teeth. Composite Resin.

REFERENCES

AQUILINO S.A,; WILLIAMS V.D,; SVARE C.W. The effect of storage solutions and mounting media on the bond strengths of a dentinal adhesive to dentin. **Dent Mater**, Iowa City, p.131-5, Jun. 1987.

BEGOSSO, M.P.; IMPARATO, J.C.P.; DUARTE, D.A. Current status of the organization of human tooth banks in dental schools in Brazil. **Ver Pós Grad**, v.8, n.1, p.23-8, 2001.

CAMPREGHER, U. B.; ARRUDA, F. Z.; SAMUEL, S. W. Means used for storing teeth in impact dental research: a systematic review. **RPG rev. pos-graduagao**, Sdo Paulo, p.107-112, Apr./Jun. 2007.

DALLANORA et al.; The effectiveness of methylparaben as a preservative for human teeth. **Final course work - Unoesc library**, 2012.

FARAH R.; DRUMMOND B.; SWAIN M.; WILLIAMS S. Linking the clinical presentation of molar-incisor hypomineralization to its mineral density. **International Journal of Paediatric Dentistry**, v.20 p.353-360, Jul. 2010.

GHERSEL E; GUEDES A.C; CIAMPONI A.L. Influence of storage mode on microleakage of deciduous teeth restored with different adhesive systems: in vitro study. **Pesqui Odontol Bras**, v.15,n.1,p.29-34,jan-mar.2001.

GIL E, BRANDÁO AL. Excipients: their applications and physico-chemical control. Editora: Pharmabooks editora, 2ed, Sdo Paulo, p.224-225, 2007.

GOODIS, H.E.; MARSHALL, Jr, G.W.; WHITE, J.M.; GEE, L.; HORNBERGER, B.; MARSHALL, S.J. Storage effects on dentin permeability and shear bond strengths. **Dent Mater**, v. 9, p. 79-84, 1993.

HALLER, B.; HOFMANN, N.; KLAIBER, N.; BLOCHING, U. Effect of storage media on microleakage of five dentin bonding agents. **Dent Mater**, v.9, p. 191-97, 1993.

IMPARATO, J.C.P. Organization and functionality of the human tooth bank (emphasis on deciduous teeth) of the Pediatric Dentistry Discipline of the School of Dentistry of the University of São Paulo. Thesis (Doctorate in Pediatric Dentistry) School of Dentistry, University of São Paulo. Sdo Paulo, p.133, 1998.

IMPARATO J.C. P.; VANZELLIM. Tooth banking: a promising idea. Stomatos, Canoas, v. 9, n. 16, p. 59-60, jan./jun. 2003.

JUNQUEIRA L. C.; CARNEIRO, J. Histologa básica, 9ª ed. Rio de Janeiro, Guanabara Koogan, 1999.

MICHELON C.; HWAS A.; BORGES M. F.; MARCHIORI, J. C.; SUSIN, A. H. Direct composite resin restorations in posterior teeth - current considerations and clinical application, **RFO**, v. 14, n. 3, p. 256-261, Sep/Dec. 2009.

MIRANDA G.E.; BUENO F.C. Human tooth bank - a bioethical analysis. **Rev. Bioét (impr.)**, p. 255, 2012.
MORERIRA L. et al, Human Tooth Bank for Teaching and Research in Dentistry. Rev. Fac. Odontol. Porto Alegre, v. 50, n. 1, p. 34-37, jan./abr., 2009.
NAKABAYASHI, N. The hybrid layer: a resin-dentin composite. **Proc. Finn. Den. Soc**, v.88, p.322-329, 1992.
NASSIF, A. C. S.; TIERI. F.; ANA DAP. A.; BOTTA. S. B.; IMPARATO J. C. P. Structuring a Human Tooth Bank. **Pesq.Odontol. Bras,** Sdo Paulo, v.17, p.70-74, May 2003. PUPO Y.M; MARTINS G.C; GOMES G.M. Influencia do tempo de armazenamento na resistencia de unido á microtrando de diferentes sistemas adesivos em dentina superficial e profunda. **Braz Dent Sci**, p.16-22,jan./jun. 2010.
SILVA, M,F; MANDARINO, F; SASSI, JF; MENEZES,de M; CENTOL,A ALB; NONAKA,T. Influence of the type of storage and the method of disinfecting extracted teeth on adhesion to tooth structure. **Revista de Odontología da Universidade Cidade de Sao Paulo**, May/Aug. 2006.
SRINIVASAN N, KAVITHA M, LOGANATHAN SC. Comparison of the remineralization potential of CPP-ACP and CPP-ACP with 900 ppm fluoride on eroded human enamel: An in situ study, p. 541, Jul. 2010.
VIEIRA, L.C.C.; BARATIERI, L.N.; LOPES, G.C.; PORTELA, R.; ANDRADE, C.A. de. Two-year clinical evaluation of composite resin restorations in posterior teeth. **JBD**, Curitiba, v. 1, n. 1, p. 72-76, jan./mar. 2002.

ARTICLE 5:

The effectiveness of methylparaben as a preservative for human teeth.

The effectiveness of methylparaben as a preservative in human teeth.

Léa Maria Franceschi DALLANORA[1] Juliana
Arcego FILIPIN[2] Juliana LANGER[3]
Fábio DALLANORA[4]
Leonardo Flores LUTHI[5]

SUMMARY

Objective: To compare whether there was a difference between storing human teeth in distilled H2O and distilled H2O plus the preservative methylparaben 0.2% in terms of enamel microhardness over a 3-month period and the effectiveness of methylparaben as a preservative for storing human teeth. **Methods**: This is an in vitro study, carried out on human teeth in the tooth bank laboratory at the University of Santa Catarina Joacaba Campus, stored in distilled H2O and a 0.2% methylparaben solution with distilled water, using a microdurometer and the depletion seeding technique for microbiological analysis. **Results:** There was no statistically significant difference in the enamel microhardness of the dental elements, both those stored in distilled water and those stored in 0.2% methylparaben solution, resulting in an overall average of 284.55 for sample Al and 302.62 for sample A2. The parabens were effective in the first 30 days, but in the subsequent samples (60 and 90 days), there was turbidity in the liquid, thus losing their inhibitory capacity. **Conclusion:** This study showed that there was no statistically significant difference in the microhardness test (Knoop) of the enamel of dental elements stored in distilled water, as well as those stored in distilled water plus methylparaben.The parabens in the first 30 days prevented bacterial and fungal proliferation, serving the purpose of preserving the liquid.

Keywords: Tooth. Storage of substances, products and materials. Distilled water

ABSTRACT

Objective: To compare whether there are differences between the storage of human teeth in distilled H 2 O in distilled H2O and more preservatives methylparaben and the hardness, during the three months and effective microbiological control. **Methods:** This work is an in vitro study performed with human teeth in laboratory tooth bank of the University of Santa Catarina in Joacaba stored in distilled water and distilled water with methylparaben and using microhardness technique of seeding by depletion of the liquid to microbiological analysis. **Results:** There was no statistically significant difference in enamel microhardness of dental elements, both stored in a solution containing distilled water and the solution stored in distilled water plus the preservative methylparaben. **Conclusion:** The present results show no statistically significant difference in enamel microhardness testing of dental elements stored in distilled water, as well as stored in distilled water plus methyl.

Key words: Tooth. Storage of substances, products and materials. distilled water

INTRODUCTION

Human tooth banks occupy a very important position within dental schools, as they are places used to store human teeth that will be used in scientific research, epidemiological tests, biological components, rehabilitation material, and even in the anatomical study of teeth by the university's academics. In addition, tooth banks seek to raise awareness among individuals about the importance of teeth as organs and their relationship to general health, as they can be used in studies for treatments, thus adding to the evolution in the view of the tooth as an integral organ of the human body (1).

However, freshly extracted teeth should be considered as a source of cross-contamination, so proper decontamination and storage allows for the maintenance of the teeth's physical properties so that they can be used in laboratory research activities, without altering the dentin substrate and offering no risk of contamination for the researcher (2).

After extraction, human teeth must be kept in a moist condition so as not to dehydrate them and alter their physical properties (1). According to Cavalcanti (3), after tooth extraction, the tooth undergoes changes, such as an increase in dentin permeability as a result of the loss of organic content from the dentin tubules, and after extraction and dental storage, there may also be interference in microtraction bond strength depending on the storage solution used.

According to Silva (4), extracted human teeth should be sent to tooth banks to be disinfected and stored in a way that does not alter their physical properties, but there is no standard substance for such procedures. However, Begosso, Imparato and Duarte (1) cite the various means used for this storage, including distilled water, which is currently the most widely used for storing human teeth, but the literature is divergent and confusing when it comes to sterilizing and disinfecting teeth.

Thus, according to Lório et al (5), further research is needed to define ways of storing teeth that do not alter and preserve dental structures, guaranteeing biosafety in the handling of specimens and leading to more concordant results in in vitro tests.

Currently, according to the literature, among the storage solutions for human teeth most often used are distilled water, 0.1% thymol, which has a preservative and disinfectant action, 0.5% chloramine T, saline solution and also freezing, which is done pure or immersed in saline solution (6).

Methylparaben is used as an antimicrobial preservative in water, food, cosmetic and pharmaceutical formulations and even toothpaste (7). It is presented as a crystalline, almost odorless and tasteless powder (8), so this study aims to use it as a method of dental storage, a solution prepared with distilled water and methylparaben (Nipagim®). Its chemical structure is illustrated in figure 1.

In research, the dental element can be subjected to various laboratory tests, one of which measures the microductivity of different dental substrates, producing a measure of the substrate's resistance to plastic deformation, which is very important for the development of new dental materials (9).

In this context, the importance of research to prove the effectiveness of methylparaben in the storage of human teeth arises, since it has antimicrobial action, investigating the possibility that it does not alter the microhardness of the enamel of dental elements.

DEVELOPMENT

The research project was submitted to and approved by the Research Ethics Committee of the Universidade do Oeste de Santa Catarina Campus de .loacaba (Process n^0 8188 /2012).

The study was carried out using 60 healthy, clean, decontaminated and non-sterile teeth from the tooth bank at UNOESC - Loacaba campus. Two samples were separated, A1 and A2 respectively, where 30 of the 60 teeth analyzed were stored in a closed container containing distilled water solution (A1), and the other sample (30 teeth) was submerged in distilled water solution plus 0.2% methylparaben preservative (A2).

Within 30 days of immersion, 10 teeth from each sample were removed from the solutions, 7 teeth were selected from this sample and chosen according to the most favorable anatomical criterion. These elements were transformed into specimens and subjected to an analysis of their physical properties using a microdurometer; the studies were carried out monthly for a period of 3 months.

During this same period, samples of the soaking liquid were collected in test tubes (every 30 days) and sown in petri dishes, with readings taken at 24 and 48 hours to check for bacterial growth.

For the microhardness test, the specimens were made as follows: the 7 teeth were sectioned in half with a carborundum disk at low speed, under cooling water, and inserted into PVC rings measuring 1 cm in height and 2 cm in diameter. Each half of the tooth was placed on a wax plate, after which the PVC was pressed into the wax so that it would be firm and the colorless self-curing acrylic resin (Clássico, Sao Paulo, SP Brazil) inside the PVC (figure 2). After acrylizing the resin, each half of the tooth was sanded on the plaster cutting machine (Soft Line) to leave the tooth surfaces flat, and then the sequence of 320, 600 and 1.200 (3M) on the Politris machine (figure 3) to make the tooth surface smooth, even and polished, allowing the analysis to be carried out using the microdurometer. The total number of specimens was 14 and 10 were analyzed. The remaining specimens were discarded and the criterion for exclusion was the smoothness of the specimen.

The microhardness of the dental element was measured using a microdurometer (figure 4) (HMV/Shimadzu Corporation- Japan- Research Laboratory, UNICAMP- Piracicaba, SP). The microhardness tester (figure 4) has a diamond penetrating tip with a pyramidal shape with a diamond base (knoop), under a static load of 100 grams for 5 seconds. When the tip is activated, it compresses the surface of the tooth, generating a diamond-shaped geometric figure.

The data was captured by the CAMS TM _WIN software (Newage testing instruments, inc.), which is a program present in the microdurometer.

The geometric shape determines the tooth's surface microhardness by measuring its longest diagonal, which is then applied to a formula to obtain the results. The microhardness value of each tooth element is given by the calculation made by the machine itself. The microhardness tester displays the result of the equation on its screen, which is the following formula

$$KHN = (C.c) / d^2$$

Thus: KNH= Knnop microhardness, C= constant 14.230, c= 500 grams and d= length of the longest diagonal of the rhombus.

For the analysis, 3 enamel endentments were carried out on each specimen.

For the microbiology tests, we used the sowing of material for analysis, which is done in various ways according to the microbiological technique. In this work, we used a collection from the bottle where the teeth are stored, one containing distilled water (A1) and the other containing a 0.2% methylparaben solution (A2).

After sowing the material, the plates containing the culture medium are incubated at the ideal temperature for the growth of mesophilic microorganisms for between 24 and 48 hours.

The bacteriological technique was used as a specific method for seeding by streaking or depletion, as this technique allows for the isolation of microorganism colonies as well as visualizing their development.

Two culture media were used to carry out the cultures: Cystine Lactose Electrolyte Deficient (CLED) Agar, which is used to promote the growth of microorganisms present in the sown material, and is a general growth medium as it allows both gram-positive and gram-negative bacteria to grow, as well as yeasts.

The second culture medium used was MacConkey Agar, which inhibits the growth of gram-positive bacteria while allowing gram-negative bacteria to grow.

RESULTS

After statistical analysis using the ANOVA method, no statistical difference was found when comparing the distilled water group (A1) and the methylparaben 0.2% solution group (A2) p=0.064, regardless of the number of months the teeth were stored in the different solutions, so the microhardness of the dental enamel remained similar in both samples, as shown in Table 1.

Equal letters show no statistical difference using the ANOVA test (P=0.05).

The ANOVA test (P=0.05) gave the following values: in the first month the teeth immersed in the distilled H2O solution plus methylparaben preservative had an average enamel microhardness of 287.64, with a standard deviation of ± 49.18, in the second month they had an enamel microhardness of 325.51 and a standard deviation of 36.31, while in the third month the average enamel microhardness of the teeth was 294.73 and the standard deviation was ±71.22.

Table 1 compares the mean dental enamel microhardness of samples A1 and A2, which showed no statistically significant mean difference between measurements (p=0.064). This result shows that there was no change in enamel microhardness in this study.

For the visual analysis of the liquids, regarding the effectiveness of methylparaben, the solution taken from bottle A1 (without preservative) showed turbidity and odor after 30 days of resting, while the liquid taken from bottle A2 (with methylparaben preservative) showed neither turbidity nor odor.

After sowing in the culture media used, bacteria and fungi were also observed in the liquid culture from flask A2, showing that this liquid was contaminated with viable microorganisms, since the preservatives do not destroy these microorganisms, but only prevent them from proliferating. This was observed in the macroscopic analysis of the Petri dishes after incubation for 24 and 48 hours at a temperature of 37° C, where bacterial colonies and fungal colonies grew in both sample A1 and sample A2.

The difference was that in sample A1, containing distilled water, the growth of microorganisms was significantly higher when compared to sample A2 containing distilled water plus methylparaben preservative, which had significantly fewer bacterial colonies, as shown in figure 5.

When the liquids were collected at 60 days, the Al liquid was completely cloudy and had a strong odor and the A2 liquid began to cloud over without having an odor, so it wasn't necessary to collect it at 90 days, since bacterial growth was evident in the previous month.

The liquids were sown on the culture media designated in the project and growth occurred in both samples, with the Al sample showing more pronounced growth. This occurred in both the 60-day samples (Al and A2) and the 90-day samples, according to the report (Annex I) presented by the Dallanora laboratory that carried out the microbiological tests.

DISCUSSION

This study evaluated the microhardness of the enamel of human teeth stored in different solutions, the teeth being clean, decontaminated and non-sterile. As well as the microhardness tests, a visual and microbiological analysis of both solutions was also carried out to determine the effectiveness of the preservative as a bacterial and fungal inhibitor.

In the analysis of dental enamel microhardness in this study, there was no statistically significant variation in enamel hardness, which, according to Donassollo (9), it is extremely important to know the physical properties of the dental element in order to understand the changes that may occur to this organ. The most important physical and mechanical properties are the modulus of elasticity, strength and dental hardness.

According to Ghersel (10), the storage medium used for human teeth can cause alterations to the tooth surface, which can be chemical and optical. In this way, the tests carried out in this study showed that the storage medium used in this study proved to be effective in terms of not altering hardness, since there was no significant difference in the dental enamel substrate.

In this study, the test of choice for dental enamel microhardness was carried out using the microdurometer, which compared the microhardness of enamel over three months, which was stored in different solutions, so according to Ghersel (10) it can be said that there is great difficulty in comparing dental microhardness values between different studies, due to the variety of tests that can be carried out for this purpose (11).

According to this study, there were no changes in the hardness of dental enamel when stored in a 0.2% methylparaben solution and in distilled water, in agreement with the study by Silva et al (4) which also showed that teeth stored only in distilled water did not undergo significant changes in microhardness (4).

The dental enamel microhardness averages found in the tests in this study, using ANOVA analysis, ranged from 245.23 to 336.15, and several studies on microhardness have shown that dental enamel has higher values than dentin (9).

The preservative of choice used for storing the teeth was a 0.2% solution of methylparaben in distilled water. Methylparaben is known commercially as nipagin®, the action of this preservative in low concentrations has a bacteriostatic and fungiostatic antimicrobial action.

Preservatives can be defined as a chemical substance whose function is to inhibit microbial growth in the product, leaving it free from degradation caused by microorganisms, be it bacteria, fungi or yeast, so this preservative solution can have a bacteriostatic and/or fungistatic function (12).

Therefore, in this study, the visual analysis of the samples (A1 and A2), more precisely the sample containing water with a concentration of 0.2% methylparaben (A2), which remained clear for more than 30 days, shows that the preservative was effective during this time, not allowing microorganisms to develop, a proliferation that would be visually evident by the cloudiness of this storage liquid.

CONCLUSION

According to the data obtained and the statistical analysis applied to the results, it can be concluded that there was no statistically significant difference (p=0.064) in the enamel microhardness test of the dental elements stored in distilled water, as well as those stored in a 0.2% methylparaben solute. In the microbiological analysis during the first 30 days of storage, the parabens prevented bacterial and fungal proliferation, serving the purpose of preserving the liquid. This lack of development of microorganisms means that the water used to preserve the teeth used in the research can be changed every 30 days of storage, but in the visual analysis of the liquid with the preservative after 60 and 90 days, (nipagim - methylparaben) showed turbidity, demonstrating that, due to the presence of microorganisms in the liquid, the preservative has lost its inhibitory capacity.

Further studies are needed with the preservative methylparaben to see if there is any alteration in the elasticity and resistance of the enamel and physical alterations in the dentin, as well as the development of a study using teeth that have been previously autoclaved and handled under aseptic conditions.

REFERENCES

1. BEGOSSO,MP; IMPARATO, JP; DUARTE, DA. Current status of the organization of human tissue banks in dental schools in Brazil. Sáo Paulo, jan./mar.2001.

2. SILVA, M,F; MANDARINO, F; SASSI, JF; MENEZES,de M; CENTOL,A ALB; NONAKA,T.Influence of the type of storage and the method of disinfection of extracted teeth on the adhesion to the dental structure. Revista de Odontologia da Universidade Cidade de Sao Paulo,2006 May-Aug.Available at: <http://www.cidadesp.edu.br/old/revista odontologia/pdf/2 maio agosto 2006/10 influencia tipo armazenamento.pdf>.

3. CAVALCANTI, AN, Santos-Daroz CB, Voltarelli FR, Lima AF, Peris AR, Marchi GM. Effect of storage periods on the bond strength of an autoconditioning adhesive system to bovine dentin. Rev Odontol UNESP. 2009.Available at:< http://rou.hostcentral.com.br/PDF/v38n4a05.pdf>.

4. SILVA, MF; MANDARINO, F; SASSI, JF; MENEZES, M; CENTOLA, ALB; NONAKA
T. Influence of the type of storage and the method of disinfecting extracted teeth on adhesion to tooth
structure. Revista de Odontologia da Universidade Cidade de Sao Paulo, 2006. May-Aug.Available at:
<http://www.cidadesp.edu.br/old/revista_odontologia/pdf/2_maio_agosto_2006/10_influencia
_storage_type.pdf>.
5TÓRIO,SL;GOMES,APM;KUBO,CH;CARNEIRO,RGF;CARNEIRO,BF;SILVA,daEG.
Evaluation of the influence of different storage media of extracted human teeth on apical marginal
infiltration. Revista de Odontologia da Universidade Cidade de Sao Paulo,2007.May-Aug.Available at:
http://www.cidadesp.edu.br/ old/revista_odontologia/pdf/5_maio_agosto_2007/avaliacao_influencia.pdf>
6.FARRET,MM;GONCALVES,TS;LIMA,EMSde;MENEZES,LMde;OSHIMA,HMS;KOCH
ENBORGER,MPMF. Influence of methodological variables on
shear bond strength. Dental Press J. Orthod. 80 v. 15, no. 1, p. 80-88,
Jan./Feb. 2010. Available at: http://www.scielo.br/pdf/dpjo/v15n1/10.pdf>.
7. Nipagin®M and Nipasol®M, Methylparaben and Propylparaben.Technical information.
8. PharmaSpecial.2004. Available at <http://www.pharmaspecial.com.br/imagens/ literatures/lit nipagin
and nipasol.pdf> GIL E, BRANDÁO AL. Excipients: their applications and physicochemical control.2 ed.
Sao Paulo;2007.224-225p.
9. DONASSOLLO,TA;ROMANO,AR;DEMARCO,FF;DELLA-BOLA,A. Evaluation of enamel and
dentin surface microhardness of bovine and human teeth (permanent and deciduous). Rev. Odonto Cienc.,
Porto Alegre, v. 22, n. 58, p. 311-316, Oct./Dec. 2007.
10. GHERSEL,ELDA;GUEDES PINTO,AC;CIAMPONI,AL. Influence of storage mode on microleakage
of deciduous teeth restored with different adhesive systems: in vitro study. Pesqui Odontol Bras
v.15,n.1,p.29-34,jan-mar.2001.
11. MAHONEY, E; HOLT,S;SWAIN,M;KILPATRICK,N. The hardness and modulus of elasticity of
primary molar teeth: an ultra-micro-indentation study. J Dent.nov.2000.
Available at <http://www.ncbi.nlm.nih.gov/pubmed/11082528> Accessed May 3, 2012.
12. Used in cosmetics. Cosmetics and perfumes. Available at:www.insumos.com.br/cosmeticos
e.../conservantes n%2044. Accessed on: August 20, 2011.

Figure 1: Chemical structure of methylparaben. Molecular formula: $C_8H_8O_3$

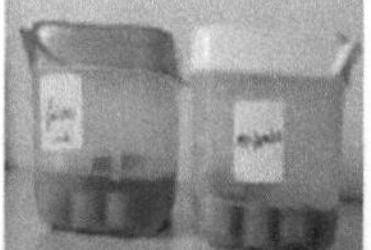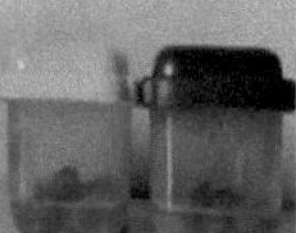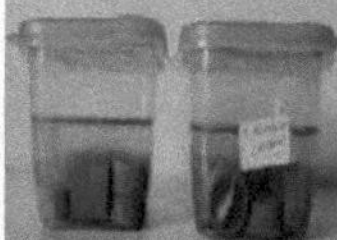

Figure 2. Containers containing samples A1 and A2 for the three months of the study.

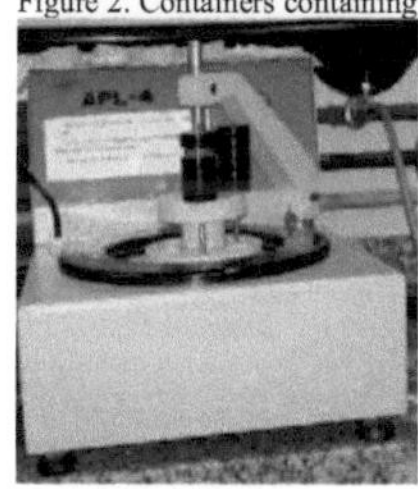

Figure 3: Polytris machine.

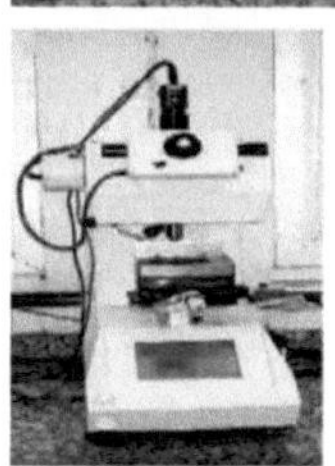

Figure 4 - Microdurometer.

	Water (A1)	Methylparaben (A2)

1	272.27±51.51 A	287.64±49.18A
2	336.15±39.60A	325.51 ±36.31 A
3	245.23±44.53 A	294.73 ±71.22A

Table 1. Shows the mean values and standard deviation between the groups in the different months of the study.

Months	Water (A1)	Methylparaben (A2)
1	272.27	287.64
2	336.15	325.51
3	245.23	294.73
Total average	248.55	302.62

Table 2. Average dental microhardness of the Ale A2 samples for each month and the total average for the three months for each sample.

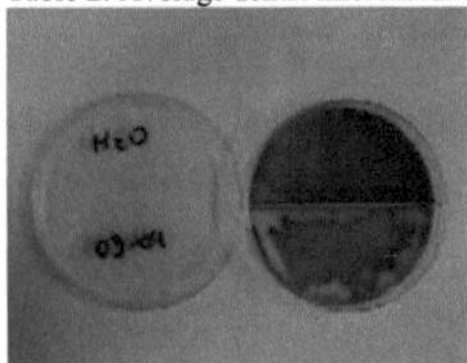

Sample Al
Figure 5.

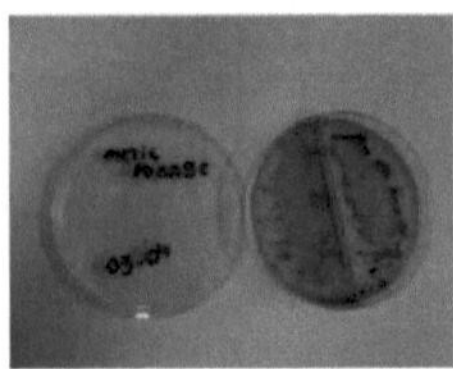

Sample A2

ARTICLE 6:

INFLUENCE OF DIFFERENT STORAGE SOLUTIONS ON ADHESION TO THE DENTAL SUBSTRATE

*

Fernanda de Lima Tissiani
Morgane Biasus
Lea Maria F. Dallanora †‡‡ §§
* ., -***
Leonardo Flores Luthi

Summary

The main aim of this study is to assess the difference between storing human teeth in distilled water and distilled water with a preservative, methylparaben, which is commercially available as Nipagin®. The study used 40 human teeth, 30 premolars and 10 molars, from the tooth bank at the University of Western Santa Catarina in Joaçaba. In this study, the physical properties of dental elements stored in different solutions were evaluated in terms of microtraction, based on adhesion to dentin using Relyx ARC resin cement, as well as the Single Bond adhesive system, between the dental substrate and the composite resin. From the results obtained, it was observed that after 30 days of storage in distilled water plus methylparaben, there were failures in the

Dentistry student at the Universidade do Oeste de Santa Catarina;

‡‡ Dentistry student at Universidade do Oeste de Santa Catarina; biasusmorgane @yahoo.com.br;

§§ Professor of Dentistry at the University of Western Santa Catarina; lea.dallanora@unoesc.edu.br;

*** Professor of Dentistry at the University of Western Santa Catarina;

leonardo.luthi@unoesc.edu.br

bond strength between the composite resin, the cement and the tooth, concluding that chemical interactions between the preservative and the dental element may have occurred.

Keywords: Tooth bank. Methylparaben. Microtraction.

1 INTRODUCTION

Teeth, like other organs in the human body, are made up of different types of tissue, including enamel, dentin, pulp and cementum; each one has a specific function, and together they are responsible for forming a fundamental structure for chewing, speaking and swallowing (JUNQUEIRA; CARNEIRO, 1999).

Dentin is a mineralized connective tissue that makes up the majority of the tooth structure, covered by enamel and cementum. This tissue houses the pulp inside and is made up of 70% hydroxyapatite, 20% organic material and 10% water (REIS; LOGUERCIO, 2007). In dentin, the influence of disinfection methods seems to be different than in enamel, since dentin is mostly composed of organic content, mainly collagen fibers (HALLER et al., 1993).

Extracted teeth are potential sources of contamination, and it is essential that the tooth bank decontaminates them. In this way, the DBH has the important function of preventing cross-infection in the indiscriminate handling of extracted teeth, since some pathogens can survive for long periods, even on dry substrates (MOREIRA et al., 2009).

Always linked to an educational institution, the Human Tooth Bank (HDB) plays an important role when it comes to research and studies in a Dentistry course, as it is legalized and provides good storage conditions for human teeth. With this, the BDH complies with the requirements of the Ethics and Research Committee, not approving research using human teeth whose origin is not proven or legalized (NASSIF, 2003).

In order to preserve human teeth in tooth banks, it is necessary to sterilize them properly and store them correctly; the literature lists different types, including: serum, dry, refrigerated and refrigerated in water, considering that some of the solutions used can interfere with the chemical and physical characteristics of dental structures (BEGOSSO; IMPARATO; DUARTE, 2001). The tooth bank is also responsible for eliminating cross-infection when these dental elements are handled incorrectly (MIRANDA; BUENO, 2012).

There is no standard substance used for the preservation and disinfection of teeth after extraction. As a result, there is a possibility that studies using similar materials on the same type of substrate will show different results due to the influence of other variables, such as the type of disinfection carried out, storage, time and type of substance used to store the tooth (SILVA et al., 2006). Thus, there is a need for standardization when it comes to storing teeth in tooth banks, but it is still difficult to find a solution that meets the needs without altering the properties of the dental element (CAMPREGHER, 2007).

Methylparaben is a paraben that has a pH of between 4-8 and has great antimicrobial action. It is a crystalline powder, almost odorless, used as a preservative in food, cosmetic and pharmaceutical formulations. The aim of this study is to use it as a dental storage method, a solution obtained with distilled water and methylparaben (Nipagin®) (GIL; BRANDÂO, 2007). According to (DALLANORA et al., 2012), the study carried out showed that there was no statistically significant difference in the enamel microhardness test of teeth stored in distilled water, as well as those stored in distilled water plus methylparaben. The parabens prevented bacterial and fungal proliferation in the first 30 days, serving the purpose of preserving the liquid. Depending on the medium in which extracted teeth are stored, this can cause chemical and optical changes to the dentin surface, affect adhesive strength, influence dentin permeability and also microleakage itself (GHERSEL; GUEDES-PINTO; CIAMPONI, 2001).

The use of dental elements *in in vitro* laboratory studies contributes to the development of new dental techniques and materials, so the existence of tooth banks is very important so that these elements can be stored and made available (FAHA et al., 2010; MANTON et al., 2010). Although *in vitro* research has improved understanding of the demineralization and remineralization process, the complex environment of the oral cavity cannot be simulated (SRINIVASAN et al., 2010).

The search for better quality dental materials has led to an increase in the number of new products appearing on the market. Therefore, in order to improve these materials and prove their effectiveness, they need to be evaluated in different laboratory tests, analyzing their clinical performance before they are used in the oral cavity (DONASSOLO et al., 2007).

Some studies show that the adhesive system factor can also interfere with the quality of the bond to dentin. This is a clinically important characteristic, since uniform behavior in the face of morphological and physiological variation of this substrate is an ideal property of an adhesive system (CLAVIJO et al., 2006).

The search for a direct material with optical characteristics similar to tooth structure resulted in the development of composite resins. As a result, composite resin has been the most intensively researched material in the last decade in order to improve certain properties and can be used in both anterior and posterior teeth (CLAVIJO etal.,2006).

In the present study, 30 premolars and 10 molars were evaluated with regard to the microtensile bond strength test between dentin and composite resin in teeth

4 stored in two different solutions, and make a comparison to see if there is a difference between storing human teeth in distilled H2O (group G1) and distilled H2O plus the preservative methylparaben (groups G2, G3 and G4) in terms of resin and dentin adhesion in microtensile tests during 30, 90 and 150 days of storage. In this context, it is important to investigate whether or not methylparaben can alter the resin's adhesion to the substrate, as seen through the microtensile test.

2 MATERIAL AND METHOD

This study was approved by the Research Ethics Committee under Opinion No. 8188. It is an analytical study with a quantitative approach and experimental research in the laboratory (*in vitro* study). It was carried out in the tooth bank of the Universidade do Oeste de Santa Catarina in Joaçaba (storage), and in the research laboratory of Preclinica II - Odontologia (microtracer test).

All the elements in the study were sterilized in an autoclave at 130 degrees for standardization, in agreement with the study by Silva et al. (2006), which concluded that the use of an autoclave seems to be the most reliable method for disinfecting teeth; the autoclave had no influence on the adhesive strength values of the teeth.

The research was carried out using a sample of 30 premolars and 10 healthy molars, stored in glass jars with lids in distilled water (Unoesc Joaçaba Distiller) and 0.2% methylparaben solution (NIPAGIN®) under refrigeration.

The 40 dental elements from the BDH complied with the biosafety storage standards suggested by Imparato (2003). The sample was divided into four groups: G1, G2, G3 and G4. Group G1 consisted of 10 teeth stored in distilled water; group G2, 10 teeth stored in distilled H2O plus methylparaben for 30 days; group G3, 10 teeth stored in distilled H2O plus methylparaben for 90 days; and group G4, 10 teeth stored in distilled H2O plus methylparaben for 150 days.

The teeth divided into groups were inserted into PVC cylinders and filled with self-curing acrylic resin (Vipi Flash Colorless), where only the dental root was inserted into the cylinder.

The dental elements were then worn down using a plaster cutter until the dentin was exposed (Photo 1); they were then sanded using a 320 e600 water sandpaper.

Photo 1 - Illustrating the process

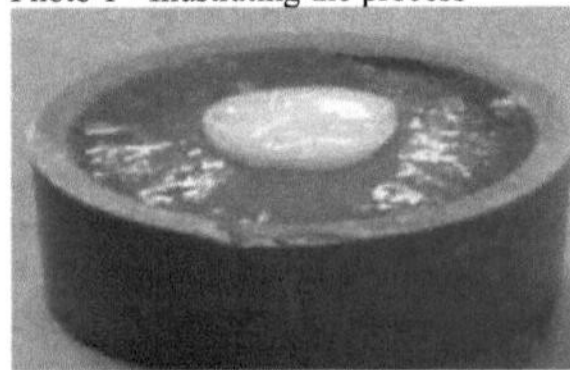

Source: the authors

Forty Opallis A2 enamel resin composite blocks were made, measuring 7 mm X 9 mm X 4 mm (Photograph 2), in 2 mm increments and photoactivated with a halogen light for 20 seconds each increment, and finally 1 minute each side, always following the same sequence of increments.

Currently, composite resin is the most widely used restorative material for direct esthetic restorations (MICHELON et al., 2009). The development of these techniques has contributed to the popularization of aesthetic restorations, especially with composite resin (VIEIRA et al., 2002). According to Clavijo (2006), an adequate restoration using the incremental composite resin technique is obtained with increments of a maximum thickness of 2 mm, followed by light-curing of each increment for 20 seconds, serving as a reference for making the resin blocks for subsequent cementing in this study.

Photo 2 - Illustrating the process

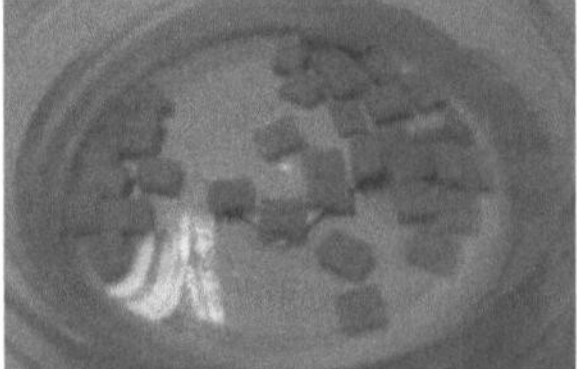

Source: the authors.
The resin blocks were sanded with a 3M 320 and 600 sandpaper on all the faces of each block and the restorations were cemented on all the teeth without differentiating between groups. First, the feather was prepared with 10% fluoride acid applied to the entire face in contact with the tooth for one minute (Photograph 3); the feather was then dried and then Silane (Prosil - FGM) was applied with a microbrush, which was rubbed on this face for 20 seconds, a jet of air was blown over it and reapplied for 20 seconds.

Photo 3 - Illustration of the process

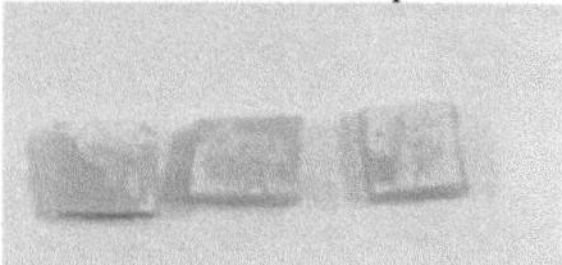

Source: the authors.

Finally, the tooth is prepared and attacked with 37% phosphoric acid (Atack tec- DentalTec) under the tooth for 15 seconds, the tooth is washed and dried for the same time, and the dentin is rewetted. A layer of Single Bond adhesive was applied using a microbrush, a distant air jet until the solvent evaporated, a new layer of adhesive was applied and the adhesive was not photoactivated (Photograph 4).

Photo 4 - Illustration of the process

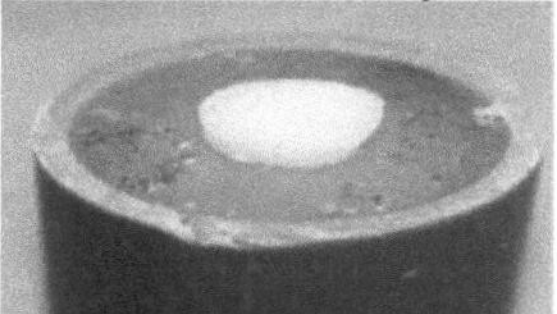

Source: the authors.

The piece was then cemented with 3M Relyx ARC. A portion of the cement was used for each tooth, and after the resin block was placed on the tooth, it was light-cured for 20 seconds on each side (Photos 5 and 6).

Photo 5 - Illustration of the process

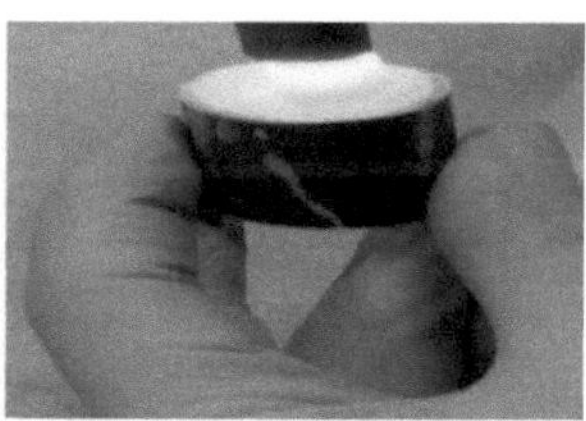

Source: the authors.
Photo 6 - Illustration of the process

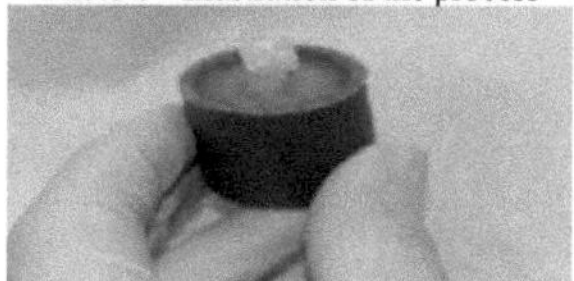

Source: the authors.
Diagram 1 - Illustration of the process

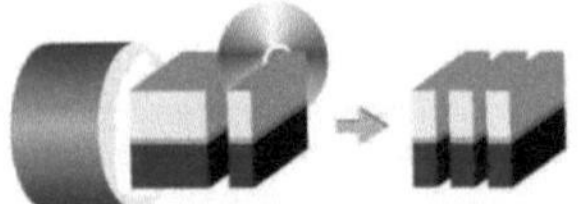

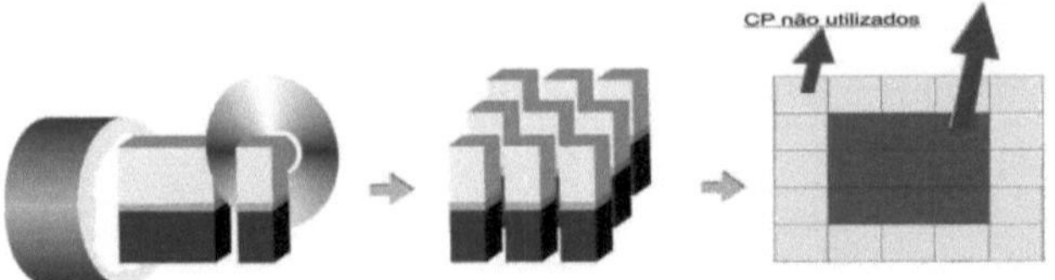

The tooth/resin set was cut on the Labcut 1010 serial cutting machine (ODEME, 2005), under constant refrigeration with water, thus obtaining specimens 1 mm wide x 1 mm high and approximately 0.5 cm long, which were used for the microtraction tests (Diagram 1).

The EMIC universal mechanical testing machine was used to carry out the microtensile test. The specimens were positioned in the device with the aid of cyanocrylate-based glue (Photo 7). A traction speed of 0.5 mm/min was used until rupture with a 100N load cell. The specimens were taken to total rupture, thus obtaining the microtensile strength values in MPa.

3 RESULTS

The non-parametric Kruskal Wallis test and Dunn's test were carried out at a significance level of 5%.

When Distilled Water (G1) was compared with Nipagin (G3 and G4) in relation to tension, a statistical difference of p=0.017 was observed and when Distilled Water (G1) was compared with Nipagin (G2), no statistical difference was found p=0.45.

Table 1 - Average values and standard deviation standard deviation for Tension (Mpa)

Group	Tension (Mpa)
G1 Distilled water	20.71±A
G2 Nipagin 9-08 (30 days)	13.49±A
G3 Nipagin 30-05 (90 days)	8.75 ±B
G4 Nipagin 15-12 (150 days)	9.33 ±B

Source: the authors.

Photo 7 - Illustration of the process

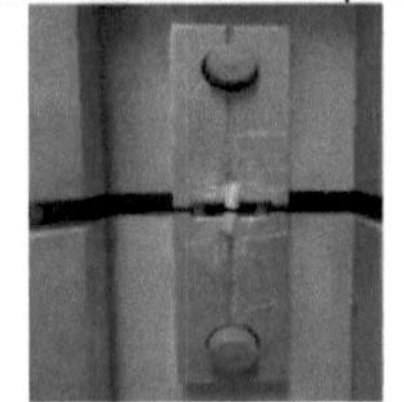

Source: Baggio et al. (2012).

In relation to strength, when Nipagin (G3 and G4) was compared to the Distilled Water group, differences of p=0.65 were found.

Table 2 - Shows mean values and standard deviation for strength

Group	Force (N)
G1 Distilled water	22.42 A
G2 Nipagin 9-08 (30 days)	13.33 A
G3 Nipagin 30-05 (90 days)	9.3 B
G4 Nipagin 15-12 (150 days)	10.10 B

Source: the authors.

4 DISCUSSION

Although laboratory tests do not faithfully reproduce the conditions that occur clinically, they represent an important analysis parameter, so the biggest challenge is to keep the resin-dentin bond stable in order to achieve longevity in restorative procedures. Therefore, various methods have been proposed to reproduce clinical situations and the oral environment, such as storage in water or other solutions. In our study, the teeth were stored in distilled water and distilled water with Nipagin as the storage medium (YAMAUTI, 2003).

Aquilino et al. (1987) evaluated the effect of the storage medium of teeth on the adhesive strength to dentin. The teeth used in the study were stored for three months in an aqueous solution of 0.9% NaCl, distilled water and a saturated solution of thymol in 0.05% distilled water. The results showed no significant difference in the values of adhesive strength to dentin, which is not the same as ours, where we found a statistical difference between groups G1, G3 and G4, with p= 0.034.

This study confirms the findings of Lorio et al. (2007), who stated that storage time is an important factor to consider, as it can generate different results. In the present study, there was no difference between the H2O G1 and Nipagin G2 30 days, while there were statistical differences between the water G1 and Nipagin G2 groups.

G3 and G4, which remained for different periods in the storage solutions.

Among the substances normally used for storage, distilled thymol water in different concentrations and physiological solution have not been shown to influence adhesive strength (AQUILINO et al. 1987; WILLIAMS; SVARE 1995; SILVA et al., 2006).

Dallanora et al. (2012) found no statistical difference in the microhardness *of the dental substrate* when comparing the distilled water group (Al) and the 0.2% methylparaben solution group (A2) p=0.064, regardless of the number of months the teeth were stored in the different solutions, This provides a basis for further research with methylparaben, which showed that there was no statistical difference between the Distilled Water (Gl) and Distilled Water and Methylparaben (G2) groups p=0.65.

In this study, there was a statistical difference of p= 0.034 when comparing the distilled water group (Gl) with distilled water and methylparaben (G3 90 days) and distilled water and methylparaben (G4 150 days), showing that there was an influence from the type of storage solution and storage time. In the study by Silva (2006), it was concluded that the solutions used to store human teeth in a tooth bank influence the changes that may occur in the dental substrate.

According to Ghersel (2001), the storage medium used for human teeth can cause alterations to the tooth surface, which can be chemical and optical, affecting adhesive strength. Thus, failures in adhesive strength were observed when comparing the Distilled Water (Gl) and Distilled Water and Methylparaben (G3 and G4) groups.

5 CONCLUSION

The solution of 0.2% methylparaben plus distilled water showed that in storage periods of less than or equal to 30 days, the adhesive strength between the substrate and the resin was not altered. However, when stored for more than 30 days, the adhesion between the composite resin and the dentin was altered, and the adhesive system or the chemical components of the resin may have interfered with the results. Further research is therefore suggested to obtain more information on the interaction between Nipagin and the dentin substrate.

Influence of different storage solutions in joining the dental substrate

Abstract

The present study aims to evaluate the difference in storage of human teeth in solution in distilled water and distilled water with preservative solution, which in this study will be Methylparaben , which presents itself as commercially Nipagin ®. For the development of the research were used 40 human teeth (premolars) teeth bank, installed at the Universidade do Oeste de Santa Catarina. We evaluated the physical properties of dental elements stored in different solutions regarding the microtensile based on the adhesion to dentin using Relyx ARC resin cement and the Single Bond between the substrate and the dental composite resin.

From the results obtained in the study, it was observed that after 30 days of storage in distilled water plus methylparaben, failure occurred in the bond strength of composite resin cement and tooth, which leads us to the conclusion that chemical interactions between the preservative and dental element may be occurring.

Keywords: Bank of teeth. Methylparaben. Microtensile.

REFERENCES

AQUILINO, S.A.; WILLIAMS, V.D.; SVARE C. W. The effect of storage solutions and mounting media on the bond strengths of a dentinal adhesive to dentin. **Dent Mater**, v.3,n. 3,p. 131-134,jun. 1987.

ARAÚJO, R. M. et al. Influence of different storage media for extracted teeth on marginal infiltration. **JBC**, v. 3, n. 14, p. 31-35, 1999.

BEGOSSO, M. P.; IMPARATO, J. C. P.; DUARTE, D. A. Current status of the organization of human tooth banks in dental schools in Brazil. **Pós Grad.**, v. 8, n. 1, p. 23-8, 2001.

CAMPREGHER, U. B.; ARRUDA, F. Z.; SAMUEL, S. W. Means used for storing teeth in impact dental research: a systemic review. **RPG**, SaoPaulo, p. 107-112, Apr./Jun. 2007.

CLAVIJO, V. G. R; SOUZA, N. C. Utilization of the self-etching adhesive system in direct composite resin restorations. **R Dental Press Estét**, Maringa, v. 3, n. 4, 2006.

DALLANORA et al. The **effectiveness of methylparaben as a preservative for human teeth**. 2012. Course Conclusion Paper (Graduation in Dentistry)-Universidade do Oeste de Santa Catarina, Joaçaba, 2012.

DONASSOLO, T. A; ROMANO, A. R. Evaluation of enamel and dentin surface microhardness of bovine and human teeth (permanent and deciduous). **Rev. Odonto Ciénc.**, Porto Alegre, v. 22, n. 58, p. 311-316, Oct./Dec. 2007.

FARAH, R. et al. Linking the clinical presentation of molar-incisor hypomineralization to its mineral density. **International Journal of Paediatric Dentistry**, v. 20 p. 353-360, July 2010.

GHERSEL, E.; GUEDES, A. C; CIAMPONI, A. L. Influence of storage mode on microleakage of deciduous teeth restored with different adhesive systems: in vitro study. **Pesqui Odontol Bras**, v. 15,n. 1,p. 29-34,jan./mar. 2001.

GIL, E.; BRANDÁO, A. L. **Excipients**: their applications and psycho-chemical control. Sao Paulo: Pharmabooks, 2007.

HALLER, B. et al. Effect of storage media on microleakage of five dentin bonding agents. **DentMater**, v. 9, p. 191-97, 1993.

IORIO, L.; GOMES, A. Evaluation of the influence of different storage media of extracted human teeth on apical marginal infiltration. **Revista de Odontologia da Universidade Cidade de Sao Paulo**, v. 19, n. 2, p. 173-180, 2007.

JUNQUEIRA, L. C.; CARNEIRO, J. **Histologa basica**. 9. ed. Rio de Janeiro: Guanabara Koogan, 1999.

MICHELON, C. et al. Direct composite resin restorations in posterior teeth: current considerations and clinical application, **RFO**, v. 14, n. 3, p. 256-261, Sept/Dec. 2009.

MIRANDA, G. E.; BUENO, F. C. Human tooth bank: a bioethical analysis. **Rev. Bioét**, p. 255, 2012.

MOREIRA, L. et al. Human teeth bank for teaching and research in Dentistry. **Rev. Fac. Odontol**. Porto Alegre, v. 50, n. 1, p. 34-37, jan./abr., 2009.

NASSIF, A. C. S. et al. Structuring a human tooth bank. **Pesq.Odontol. Bras**, Sao Paulo, v. 17, p. 70-74, 2013.

ODEME DENTAL RESEARCH. 2005. Available at: <http://www.odeme.com.br/empresa.php>. Accessed on: May 15, 2013.

REIS, Alessandra; LOGUERCIO, Alessandro Dourado. **Direct dental materials:** from fundamentals to clinical application. Sao Paulo: Santos, 2007.

SILVA, M. F. et al. Influence of the type of storage and the method of disinfection of extracted teeth on the adhesion to the dental structure. **Revista de Odontologia da Universidade Cidade de Sao Paulo**, 2006.

SRINIVASAN, N.; KAVITHA, M.; LOGANATHAN, S. C. Comparison ofthe remineralization potential of CPP-ACP and CPP-ACP with 900 ppm fluoride on eroded human enamel: an in situ study. **Arch Oral Biol.**, v. 55, n. 7, p. 541-544, jul. 2010.

VIEIRA, L.C.C. et al. Two-year clinical evaluation of composite resin restorations in posterior teeth. **JBD**, Curitiba, v. 1,n. 1,p. 72-76,jan./mar. 2002.

YAMAUTI, M. et al. Degradation of resin-dentin bonds using NaOCl storage. **Dent Mater**, v. 19, n. 5, p. 399-405, 2003.

ARTICLE 8:

INFLUENCE OF STORAGE TIME OF HUMAN TEETH ON ADHESION TO THE DENTAL SUBSTRATE

Gessica Esteves[10] Léa Maria F. Dallanora[11]

SUMMARY

This study evaluated the difference between storing human teeth for 24 months, 12 months and 3 months in a sterile distilled water solution in unrefrigerated bottles, and a control group of human teeth stored for 3 months in a distilled water solution under refrigeration. The study used 40 molars from the tooth biobank at the Universidade do Oeste de Santa Catarina - Campus Joaçaba. The physical properties of the dental elements were observed with regard to microtraction, based on the dentin adhesion of the Single Bond adhesive system between dentin substrate and composite resin. In the light of the research carried out, it was possible to observe that over time the values showed a drop in adhesion properties, but no statistical difference was found between the groups studied. This proves that teeth stored for 3 months to 24 months can be used in scientific research into dentin adhesion, without interfering in the final results.
Keywords: Microtraction. Adhesion. Biobank of teeth.

1INTRODUCTION

Tooth banks and biobanks are non-profit organizations linked to a university or institution, providing study material for students in academic life or for researchers. MIRANDA, BUENO (2012), report that, "In Brazil, the first human tooth bank was that of the pediatric dentistry department at the University of São Paulo School of Dentistry (FO-USP), in 1992". In 1997, with the formulation of the Transplant Law in Brazil, teeth began to be known as organs, raising ethical questions about the illegal trade in human teeth (GOMES et al., 2013).

Currently, for the use of these teeth, most Research Ethics Committees (RECs) require the researcher to provide proof of the origin of the teeth or a free and informed consent form signed by the donor, through which the donor authorizes and legalizes the donation (GOMES et al., 2013). Thus, teeth donated to biobanks and tooth banks are always accompanied by the free and informed consent of the donors (FREITAS et al., 2010).

The use of human teeth for research, laboratory or clinical procedures must respect ethical and legal aspects, and researchers, educators, students and the general public need to be concerned about the proper procedures with which these organs are treated (VANZELLI; IMPARATO, 2003).

Always linked to a teaching institution, the tooth bank plays an important role when it comes to research and studies at a dental university. Because it is legalized and provides good storage conditions for human teeth, the tooth bank complies with the requirements of the CEP, since it does not approve research using human teeth whose origin is not proven or legalized (NASSIF et al., 2003). The establishment of tooth banks in educational institutions is essential to enable research and technological innovations using human teeth (NASSIF et al., 2003). A tooth bank linked to dental courses gradually reduces the chances of cross-infection and organizes the use of these dental elements in research and extension projects (POLETTO et al.,

---

[10] Dentistry undergraduate student, Universidade do Oeste de Santa Catarina; esteves.ge@hotmail.com

[11] Specialist in Pediatric Dentistry at the Bauru Regional Dentistry Association of São Paulo; Professor of Dentistry at the Universidade do Oeste de Santa Catarina; lea.dallanora@unoesc.edu.br

2010).

After being extracted from the oral cavity, dental elements are considered organs and must be handled correctly to prolong their useful life, as they will be used for research, either by students at the university or by researchers from other schools (DALLANORA et al., 2015). They must be kept in a humid condition so as not to dehydrate them and alter their physical properties. Many media are used for this storage, including distilled water, which is currently the most widely used for storing human teeth in tooth banks, as in the studies by: BEGOSSO; IMPARATO; DUARTE, 2001, CESCA; DALLANORA; LUTHI, 2014, DALLANORA et al., 2015. The solutions used to store human teeth in tooth banks, as well as the length of time they have been immersed, influence possible changes in the dental substrate (SILVA et al., 2006).

Teeth are a major source of contamination, and it is essential for tooth banks and biobanks to decontaminate them correctly, preventing cross-infection. However, it is also essential to maintain their chemical, physical and mechanical properties, so that there are no biases in the research carried out on them (MOREIRA et al., 2009).

According to the study carried out by CESCA; DALLANORA; LUTHI, (2014) distilled water plus methylparaben had a significant loss of adhesion of the dental substrate to the composite resin when compared to storage in distilled water. There is a clear need for standardization when it comes to storing teeth in tooth banks, but it is difficult to obtain a liquid medium that meets these needs without altering the properties of the dental organ (MOREIRA et al., 2009).

When the organ arrives at the tooth bank, it goes through a series of disinfection procedures so that it can be stored, as the tooth after extraction is a potential source of contamination and cross-infection, so it must be handled in accordance with biosafety standards (MOREIRA et al., 2009). The action of decontamination agents or the storage method should not modify important characteristics of dental tissue, such as dentin bond strength and microleakage (MOREIRA et al., 2009). In dentin, the influence of disinfection methods may be different than in enamel, since there is a greater organic content represented mainly by collagen fibers (VINHOLES, FERNANDES, RITZEL, 2001).

According to Silva et al. (2006, p. 176),

> With regard to experiments aimed at testing the mechanical properties of various adhesive restorative materials on dental tissues, maintaining the normal condition of this substrate is essential in order to achieve the closest possible reproduction of the situations that occur in the oral cavity.

In this context, the importance of research to prove how long teeth can be stored without altering their physical properties arises, evaluating the tooth/resin adhesion capacity using Single Bond adhesive.

2 MATERIALS AND METHODS

This is an analytical study with a quantitative approach and an experimental investigation in the laboratory (*in vitro* study). The study was carried out in the laboratory of the Tooth Biobank of the Universidade do Oeste de Santa Catarina in Joaçaba, in the preclinical research laboratory II - Dentistry (microtraction test). This study was approved by the CEP under number 2.094.259.

The study used 40 molars from the Human Teeth Biobank (BDH) at UNOESC - Joaçaba campus, which were cleaned and sterilized according to biosafety standards. Four groups of samples were studied, G1, G2, G3 and G4, as follows: the first group contained a sample of 10 analyzed teeth, stored submerged in a distilled water solution under refrigeration (G1) for 3 months, with the storage solution being changed every 8 days; the second group contained a sample of 10 teeth stored in a sealed glass container, containing sterile distilled water solution (G2) for 3 months, third group with a sample of 10 teeth stored in a sealed glass container containing sterile distilled water solution (G3) for 12 months, fourth group with a sample of 10 teeth stored in a sealed glass container containing sterile distilled water solution (G4) for 24 months.

The coronal part of the enamel was removed, leaving only the dentin, in order to make the resin block with a size of 2 mm, which was standardized on all the teeth without differentiating between groups. First, the tooth was sprayed with 37% phosphoric acid for 30 seconds, rinsed and dried for the same time. A layer of Single Bond adhesive (3M - Sumaré - Sao Paulo) was applied with a microbrush, then a jet of air was applied from a distance until the solvent evaporated, then another layer of adhesive was applied, then a jet of air was applied and the adhesive was polymerized for 10 seconds (Gnatus Optilight Plus light-curing device). The restoration was then made with Opallis A2 enamel composite resin (FGM- Joinville - Santa Catarina), light-cured for 20 seconds using the same technique as the previous work, with each increment of resin, and then over-cured for 40 seconds on all sides of the tooth. The tooth/resin set was cut on a serial cutting machine under constant cooling with water, thus obtaining 15 specimens from each group measuring 1mm wide x 1mm high and approximately 0.5cm long, which were used for the microtraction tests.

In the microtensile test carried out on the universal mechanical testing machine, the specimens were positioned in the device with the aid of cyanocrylate-based glue (Super Bonder Gel, Loctite Ltda., Piracicaba, SP, Brazil) and a traction speed of 0.5 mm/min was used until rupture with a 100N load cell. The specimens were taken to total rupture, thus obtaining the microtensile strength values in MPa.

After obtaining and tabulating the results, they were subjected to ANOVA statistical tests.

4-Results

After tabulating the data, we obtained the average maximum stress values in Mpa and the standard deviation for each group. It was possible to observe that over time the values showed a decrease in adhesion properties, but no statistical difference was found between the groups studied (table 1). After performing the one-factor ANOVA test in the SPSS program, the P value found was ($p=0.132$).

Table 1. Shows the average values in Mpa and the standard deviation for each study group.

Equal capital letters between the groups show no statistical significance using the ANOVA test with a significance level of 0.05%.

At the time of fracture, the different patterns were evaluated, and in all groups the "Adhesive" fracture pattern was the one with the highest percentage values, which is a corroborating result for our study, as it means that the bond strength is lower than the strength of the tooth or resin. The cohesive and mixed fracture forms had a lower percentage, again proving that the quality of the dental substrate used in the resin adhesion is maintained.

Table 2 Shows the percentage values of the different fracture patterns.

Group	Average in Mpa
G1 (control)	33,8±(13,33)A
G2	31,5±(10,4)A
G3	30,8 ± (8,89) A
G4	30,4±(11,34)A

Group	Adhesive	Cohesive	Mixed
1	60%	30%	10%
2	65%	20%	15%
3	70%	25%	5%

4	80%	20%	0%

5- Discussion

This study evaluated the influence of storage time on the bond strength of an adhesive system and composite resin to the dental tissue of human teeth, using the groups of teeth Gl, G2, G3 and G4. The teeth were cleaned, decontaminated and sterile, in accordance with what is recommended in the literature by Silva in 2006. The microtensile strength test, originally developed by Cavalcanti et al. in 2009, was used to assess bond strength in small areas of dental substrates, as was duplicated in the present study.

All the elements in the study were sterilized in an autoclave at 30°C to ensure homogeneity. This agrees with the study by Silva et al. (2006), who concluded that the use of an autoclave seems to be the most reliable method for disinfecting teeth, with no influence on the adhesive strength values of the teeth, justifying the minimal loss of adhesion between Gl and G2, where Gl was sterilized only once, and G2 was autoclaved twice, following the SOPs of the UNOESC Human Teeth Biobank.

The way in which the teeth are stored and the method of disinfection can have major influences on the results, and the present study used only autoclave sterilization and storage with distilled water, as both methods are recommended in the literature, in the studies by BEGOSSO; IMPARATO; DUARTE, 2001, CESCA; DALLANORA; LUTHI, 2014, DALLANORA et al.,2015.

Several factors can alter adhesion strength, such as storage time, the solution used for storage and the disinfection technique, which led us to carry out the study by testing the storage time of teeth stored only in distilled water. Silva et al., 2006 reported in their study that the type of storage solution can affect dentin permeability and has a major influence on dentin adhesion, with distilled water, thymol and saline solution obtaining the best results.

In this study there was no significance between storage time and adhesive capacity, as the time increased from 3 months to 24 months there was little variation in adhesive properties, with no statistically significant results. This is in line with the study by Martins (2008) where he reported that bond strength gradually decreases with storage time, but nothing significant, and with the research by Calvacanti et al., (2009) where in their study there was no statistical difference between the groups in terms of storage time.

This study showed that teeth cleaned by scraping and autoclaving and stored in distilled water in sealed bottles for a long period of time did not lose their physical adhesion properties, with strength results of 31.5 Mpa in G2 to 30.4 Mpa in G4, while the control group G1 had a strength of 33.8 Mpa, which can be used for research without resulting in bias at the end of the study. This agrees with the researchers Martins (2008) and Calvacanti et al. (2009), who concluded that storage time does not affect the physical properties of teeth.

6- Conclusion

This study showed that teeth stored according to the Standard Operating Procedures of the Human Teeth Biobank at UNOESC retain their physical adhesion properties, with a non-statistically significant decrease in adhesion over a storage period of up to 24 months. The teeth stored in the BDH can therefore be used for research into dentin adhesion with dental materials. However, further studies with longer storage times are suggested in order to prove how long the teeth maintain their physical adhesive properties.

ABSTRACT

The present study evaluated the difference in the storage of human teeth at 24 months, 12 months and 3 months in sterile distilled water solution, and the control group of 3 month human teeth stored in distilled water solution on refrigeration. For the development of the research 40 molars of the Biobank for Teeth installed at the University of the West of Santa Catarina, Joaçaba, were used. The physical properties of dental elements with respect to microtraction were observed based on the adhesion strength of the dentine of the Single Bond adhesive system, between dentine substrate and composite resin. In view of the research, it was possible to observe that over time the values showed a decrease in the adhesion properties, but no statistical difference was found between the studied groups. Proving that teeth stored from 3 months to 24 months can be used in scientific research, not interfering in the final results.

Keywords: Microtraction. Adhesion. Biobank for Teeth.

7-REFERENCES

BEGOSSO, M.P.; IMPARATO, J.C.P.; DUARTE, D.A. Current status of the organization of human tooth banks in dental schools in Brazil. Ver Pós Grad, v.8, n.1, p.23-8, 2001.

CAVALCANTI, N. A.; DAROZ, S. B. C.; VOLTARELLI, R. F.; LIMA, F. A.; PERIS, R. A.; MARCHI, M. G. Effect of storage periods on the bond strength of an autoconditioning adhesive system to bovine dentin, Rev Odontol UNESP, Araraquara, v. 38, n. 4, p. 222-27,jul./ago. 2009.

CESCA, G.; DALLANORA, M. F. L.; LUTHI, F. L. Influence of different storage solutions on the bond strength of an adhesive system and composite resin to dental enamel. Rev. Açao Odontologia, v.5 n.1 2014.

DALLANORA, J. F.; DALLANORA, F. M. L.; ESTEVES, C. G.; CHIOCCA, S. R.; RAMOS, C. A. Human tooth bank: conditioning of dental elements. Editora UNOESC. 2015.

FREITAS, A. D. B. A.; CASTRO, L. D. C.; SETT, J. S. G.; BARROS, M, L.; MOREIRA, N. A.; MAGALHÄES, S. C. Use of extracted teeth in dental research published in Brazilian journals with free online access: a study from the perspective of bioethics, Arq. Odontol. vol.46 no.3 Belo HorizonteJul./Sept. 2010.

GOMES, M. G.; GOMES, M. G.; PUPO, M. Y.; GOMES, M. M. O.; SCHMIDT, M. L.; KOZLOWSKI, J. A. V. The use of human teeth: ethical and legal aspects: RGO, Rev. gaúch. odontol. (Online) vol.61 supl.1 Porto Alegre Jul./Dec. 2013.

MARTINS, C. G. Effect of water storage on the bond strength of different dentin adhesion approaches, Ponta Grossa, 2008.

MIRANDA, G. L; BUENO, F. C; Human tooth banking, a bioethical analysis. Rev bioét (impr.) 2012; 20 (20): 255-66.

MOREIRA, L; GENARI, B; STELLO, R; COLLARES, F. M; SAMUEL, W. M. Banco de Dentes Humanos para o Ensino e Pesquisa em Odontologia. Rev. Fac. Odontol. Porto Alegre, v. 50, n. 1, p. 34-37, jan./abr., 2009.

NASSIF, Alessandra C.S; TIERI, Fabio; ANA, Patricia, da Aparecida; BOTTA, Sergio, B; IMPARATO, José, C,P. Structure of a Human Tooth Bank. Pesqui Odontol Bras,2003.

POLETTO, M. M; MOREIRA, M; DIAS, M. M; LOPES, M. G. K; LAVORANTI O. J; PIZZATTO, E. Banco de dentes humanos: perfil sociocultural de um grupo de doadores RGO, Porto Alegre, v. 58, n.1, p. 91-94,jan./mar. 2010.

SILVA, M. F; MANDARINO, F; SASSI, J. F; MENEZES, M; CENTOLA, A. L. B; NONAKA, T. Influence of the type of storage and the method of disinfection of extracted teeth on adhesion to the dental structure. Revista de Odontologia da Universidade Cidade de São Paulo: May-Aug; 18(2)175-80 2006.

VANZELLI, M.; RAMOS, D.L.P.; IMPARATO, J.C.P. Valuing the tooth as an organ. In: IMPARATO, J.C. Banco de Dentes Humanos. Curitiba: Editora Maio, ch.2, p.31-7, 2003.

VINHOLES, M. A. I. J.; FERNANDES, C. D.; RITZEL, F. I. Banco de dentes humanos no curso de odontologia da ulbra - campus torres, Rio Grande do Sul, 2001.

ARTICLE 9

STUDY OF MICROBIOLOGICAL CONTROL AND MICROHARDNESS OF TEETH STORED IN THE UNOESC HUMAN TEETH BIOBANK JOAÇABA

BANDEIRA, Ana Paula[12]
CHIOCCA, Rosane Siepmann[13]
DALLANORA, Léa Maria Franceschi[14]
DALLANORA, Fábio José[15]

SUMMARY

The Human Teeth Biobank at UNOESC Joaçaba is an extremely important space within the University for the Dentistry course. It is used for storing human teeth, which should be considered a source of cross-contamination, so correct decontamination and storage allow the physical properties of the teeth to be maintained and the risk of contamination to be reduced. The aim of the study was to assess the quality of the microbiological control of teeth stored in the BDH, according to its adopted SOPs, its real effectiveness and whether the method does not influence the physical characteristics of dental elements such as microhardness. The work was carried out by means of an in vitro study with human teeth in the BDH laboratory, stored in distilled H2O and sealed hermetically, using a microdurometer and the depletion seeding technique for microbiological analysis. The results showed that the samples evaluated were free of contamination and, statistically, there were only changes in the microhardness of teeth stored for two years. It can be seen that the teeth stored in the BDH at UNOESC are free from contamination and can be used safely in laboratory research activities. With regard to microhardness, it was found that the teeth that underwent the greatest variation in physical characteristics were those from G5, making it impossible to use them in microhardness-related

[12] Dentistry undergraduate student, Universidade do Oeste de Santa Catarina; aniiiinhaa_pb@hotmail.com
[13] Dentistry undergraduate student, Universidade do Oeste de Santa Catarina; chiocca.familia@hotmail.com
[14] Specialist in Pediatric Dentistry at the Bauru Regional Dentistry Association of São Paulo; Professor of Dentistry at the Universidade do Oeste de Santa Catarina; lea.dallanora@unoesc.edu.br
[15] Specialist in Clinical Analysis at AVM Faculdade Integrada; Professor of Dentistry at Universidade do Oeste de Santa Catarina; fabio.dallanora@unoesc.edu.br

research. This shows that the teeth stored in the BDH at UNOESC can be used in various scientific research laboratory activities.

Keywords: Tooth biobank. Microbiology. Microhardness. Tooth.

1INTRODUCTION

The Biobanco de Dentes Humanos (BDH) is a non-profit institution linked to the Universidade do Oeste de Santa Catarina - UNOESC Joaçaba and its purpose is to store the dental elements provided in a correct and sterile manner, which will be used specifically for research and pre-clinical laboratory training for the students of the Dentistry course. They must also ensure the integrity of the components of the Biobank, academics, teachers and researchers when handling these elements and, to this end, they must take care to sterilize and/or disinfect the teeth to eliminate cross-infection when handling them after exodontia (IMPARATO, 2003).

The dental elements stored in UNOESC's Biobank of human teeth come from cessation, collection from private clinics, health centers and the institution's dental clinics. This is due to extensive awareness-raising work carried out among academics, professionals in the field and the community. It is also up to the tooth banks to raise awareness among individuals about the importance of teeth as an organ and their relationship with health in general and that they are subject to the Brazilian Transplant Law (Law 9434 of February 4, 1997), so it is necessary to know the origin of each tooth donated to these institutions (IMPARATO, 2003).

Teeth are used by academics and other professionals in the field to carry out research work and, to this end, great care must be taken to sterilize them, as well as maintaining the integrity and physical characteristics of the stored elements. They must be considered infectious and the infectious agents associated with them must be eliminated, with minimal structural alterations and changes in the biomechanical properties of the tissues being desirable, or ideally, that these do not occur during this process (BRAUER et al., 2008; MOSCOVICH et al., 1999; WHITE et al., 1994).

Normally, teeth that have been extracted are stored in some kind of solution after being extracted and before being sterilized. However, the effect of storage solutions and sterilization on enamel and dentin is unclear (LEE et al, 2007).

According to Silva et al. (2006), extracted human teeth should be sent to tooth banks to be disinfected and stored in a way that does not alter their physical properties, but there is no standard substance for these procedures. However, the scientific literature mentions different means of storage and substances used, such as distilled water and the same for sterilization, which causes some confusion and doubts about which method to adopt (BEGOSSO, IMPARATO and DUARTE, 2001).

According to Nassif (2003), dental elements should only be handled by individuals wearing personal protective equipment (PPE) in order to avoid cross-contamination. The preparation, selection and methods of disinfecting/sterilizing teeth can vary according to the research and, above all, the purpose for which the teeth are intended.

The use of extracted elements in in situ experiments contributes to the development of new techniques and dental materials. Teeth should be considered a potential source of cross-infection, so efficient decontamination methods should be adopted before use (FARRET et al., 2001).

In addition to the storage conditions that allow their properties to be maintained, the storage solutions for human teeth that are most often used include distilled water, 0.1% thymol, which has a preservative and disinfectant action, 0.5% chloramine T, saline solution and also freezing, which is carried out pure or immersed in saline solution (FARRET et al., 2001).

The microhardness of dentin or enamel is considered to depend on the amount of mineral content in its composition (PASHLEY et. al., 1985; DE-DEUS et. al., 2006; DEDEUS et. al. 2008) and its determination generally provides indirect evidence of mineral loss or gain in dental hard tissues (PATIL. UPPIN, 2011; ARENDS. TEN BOS, 1992).

In this context, the importance of research to prove the effectiveness of the standard operating procedures adopted by the Tooth Biobank regarding the storage and storage of teeth and especially whether their physical properties are preserved arises.

2 MATERIAL AND METHOD

This study was submitted to and approved by the Ethics and Research Committee of the Universidade do Oeste de Santa Catarina de Joaçaba (Opinion No.⁰ 2.092.871).

The microbiological research was carried out using 17 (seventeen) tooth vials, 15 (fifteen) of which containing hygienic teeth, which were cleaned, sterilized, immersed in distilled water, sealed hermetically and sterilized again, stored inside the BDH in a dry place without refrigeration, dating from 1 (one) month before the start of the research to 2 (two) years in storage. The control group used 2 (two) bottles containing clean teeth which were only cleaned and decontaminated.

For seeding by exhaustion, the streaking or exhaustion technique (bacteriological technique) was used, as it allows not only the visualization of the development of colonies, but also their isolation.

Three media were used for the cultures: *MacConkey Agar*, which inhibits the growth of gram-positive bacteria and allows the growth of gram-negative bacteria. The second medium was *Cystine Lactose Electrolyte Deficient (CLED) Agar*, which is used to promote the growth of microorganisms present in the sown material, and is a general growth medium as it allows both gram-positive and gram-negative bacteria to grow. The third was *Difco Mitis Salivarius Agar*, which is used to identify specific oral bacteria (*Streptococcus mitis, Streptococcus salivarius and Enterococcus*); these organisms are involved in cariogenesis and infective endocarditis.

After sowing the material (soaking liquid), the Petri dishes containing the culture medium were incubated in a greenhouse at 36.5°C (±1°C) and read after 24 and 48 hours to check for the growth of microorganisms.

For the microhardness test, the specimens were made as follows: we selected 50 teeth and divided them into groups of 10 to facilitate evaluation and control of the data obtained: G1 - Control Group (extracted teeth not filled); G2 - 3 months (20.05.17); G3 - 6 months (24.11.16); G4 - 1 year (01.12.16) and G5 - 2 years (15.04.15) and specifically the group of upper and/or lower incisors. Each tooth was fixed with sticky wax in PVC rings measuring 2 cm in height and 2 cm in diameter, with the inside filled with colorless self-curing acrylic resin (photo 1) and then all sanded using a Polytris machine (photo 2) with water sandpaper using 320, 600 and 1200 grit (3M), in order to obtain a flat, smooth and regular surface to facilitate analysis using the microdurometer.

Photo 1 - Test specimens
Photo 2 - Polytris machine

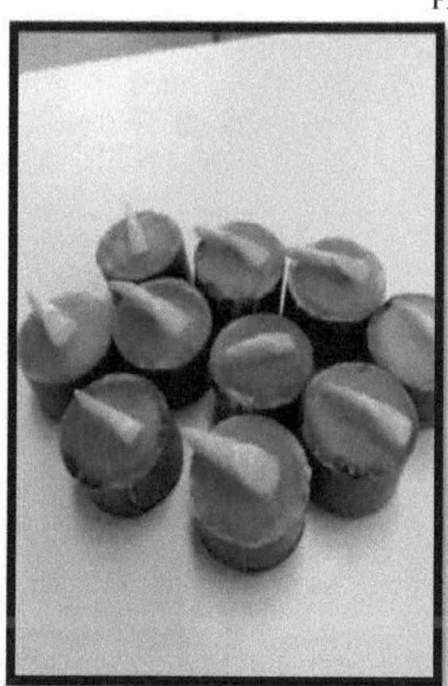

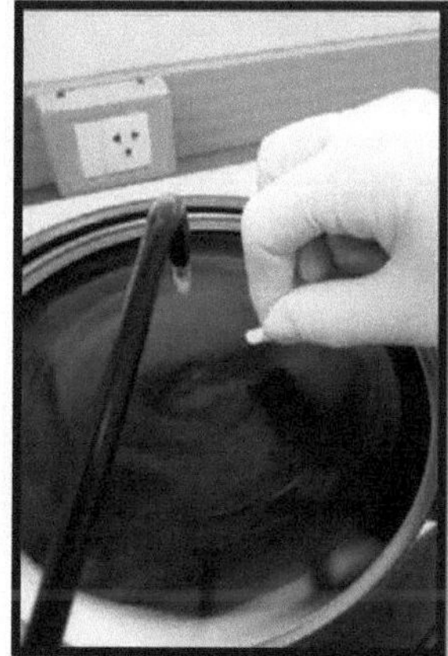

Source: the authors

RESULTS

In the visual analysis of the liquids (distilled water) contained in the bottles submitted for evaluation, those stored for two years showed no turbidity of the liquid and no odor when opened, while the control group showed turbidity and a slight odor.

After being sown in the culture media used, bacteria were seen to grow in the liquid in the Petri dishes of the control group (photo 3), visually showing that this flask contained liquid contaminated by microorganisms and that this growth occurred after being incubated for the specified time at a temperature of 36.5° C (±1°C).

Photo 3- Growth of microorganisms
Photo 4- No microorganism growth

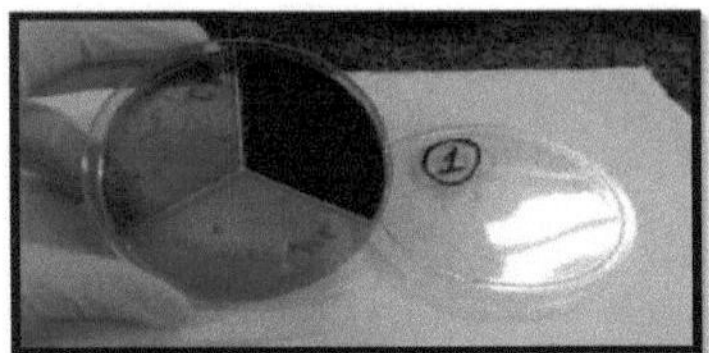

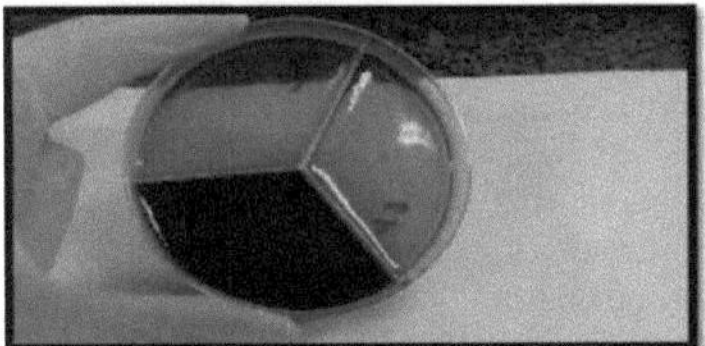

Source: the authors.

All the remaining bottles that were stored according to the BDH's SOPs after sowing in the Petri dishes (photo 4) showed no bacterial growth.

As for the microhardness tests, the data was tabulated in an Excel® spreadsheet. Then, using the SPSS® 21 program (Statistical Package for the Social Sciences), descriptive statistics were performed and compared between the groups. To verify the difference between the groups, the ANOVA test was performed followed by Tukey's post-test. The significance level was 0.05.

Table 1 shows the average values obtained for Knoop microhardness. A significant difference was found when comparing the control groups (G1) 233.40, 3 months (G2) 220.40, 6 months (G3) 160.40 and 1 year (G4) 179.90 to the group that was kept sterilized for 2 years (G5) 69.10, so the microhardness of the dental enamel did not remain similar in both samples.

Table 1- Average microhardness of the groups studied.

Group				
Control (G1)	3 months (G2)	6 months (G3)	1 year (G4)	2 years (G5)
Average	Average	Average	Average	Average
233,40	220,40	160,40	179,90	69,10

Source: the authors

The ANOVA test followed by Tukey's post-test showed that there was a statistically significant difference when comparing the groups: Control x 6 months - p=0.004: Microhardness was higher in the control group; Control x 2 years - p =0.000: Microhardness was higher in the control group; 6 months x 3 months - p =0.027: Microhardness was higher in the 1-year group; 6 months x 2 years - p =0.000: Microhardness was higher in the 6-month group; 1 year x 2 years - p =0.000: Microhardness was higher in the 1-year group; 2 years x 3 months - p =0.000: Microhardness was higher in the 3-month group. The treated group that obtained the best result in the microhardness test was the 3-month post-treatment group (mean = 220.4) as shown in Table 2. ...

Table 2- Post Hoc Tests.

Multiple comparisons
Dependent variable: Evaluation

Tukey HSD						
(I) Group	(J) Group	Average difference (I-J)	Standard model	Sig.	95% confidence interval	
					Limit lower	Upper limit
Control	3 months	13,000	19,397	,962	-42,12	68,12
	6 months	73,000*	19,397	,004	17,88	128,12
	1 year	53,500	19,397	,061	-1,62	108,62
	2 years	164,300*	19,397	,000	109,18	219,42
3 months	Controle	-13,000	19,397	,962	-68,12	42,12
	6 months	60,000*	19,397	,027	4,88	115,12
	1 year	40,500	19,397	,243	-14,62	95,62
	2 years	151,300*	19,397	,000	96,18	206,42
6 months	Controle	-73,000*	19,397	,004	-128,12	-17,88

(I) Group	(J) Group	Average difference (I-J)	Standard model	Sig.	Limit lower	Upper limit
	3 months	-60,000*	19,397	,027	-115,12	-4,88
	1 year	-19,500	19,397	,852	-74,62	35,62
	2 years	91,300*	19,397	,000	36,18	146,42
1 year	Controle	-53,500	19,397	,061	-108,62	1,62
	3 months	-40,500	19,397	,243	-95,62	14,62

	6 months	19,500	19,397	,852	-35,62	74,62
	2 years	110,800*	19,397	,000	55,68	165,92
2 years	Control e	-164,300*	19,397	,000	-219,42	-109,18
	3 months	-151,300*	19,397	,000	-206,42	-96,18
	6 months	-91,300*	19,397	,000	-146,42	-36,18
	1 year	-110,800*	19,397	,000	-165,92	-55,68

*. The mean difference is significant at the 0.05 level. Source: the authors

3 DISCUSSION

Adequate methods of sterilizing the dental substrate are necessary if extracted teeth are to be used in laboratory research and, above all, in in situ tests, since potentially pathogenic microorganisms can be present in the tooth even if it has been cleaned under running water (PAGNINO et al.,1985). Such methods should promote sterilization without introducing significant changes in the properties of the dental element.

The aim of this study was to use a method that effectively sterilizes dental substrates, not just disinfects them, and to store them without the need for refrigeration, just by keeping them in a cool, clean place.

In this way, 15 jars containing the specimens stored over a period of 30 days (02.06.17) to 2 years (17.02.15) of storage, in which the following standard operating procedures were adopted: the first procedure is to autoclave the teeth (photos 4 and 6); the second procedure is to select the teeth, classifying them as clean, restored, decayed and for disposal due to their inability to be used in research (photo 7); the third procedure is cleaning to remove adhered organic matter (photo 8); the fourth procedure is sorting by dental group, making it easier when requested for research; the fifth procedure is storing the teeth in 50 and 100 ml clear glass jars, immersed in distilled water and closed with a rubber lid and aluminum seal (photo 9); the sixth procedure is autoclaving these jars, keeping the teeth in a sterile environment (photo 10). After the procedures, the vials are stored in a cupboard with identification of the dental element, quantity and date of sterilization (photo 11). Except for the control group, which only underwent cleaning and decontamination and was stored in vials submerged in distilled water. All the teeth have their origin and destination documented (photo 12).

Photo 5- Cleaning Photo 6- Autoclaving Photo 7- Pre-selection Photo 8- Chapel (Cleaning)

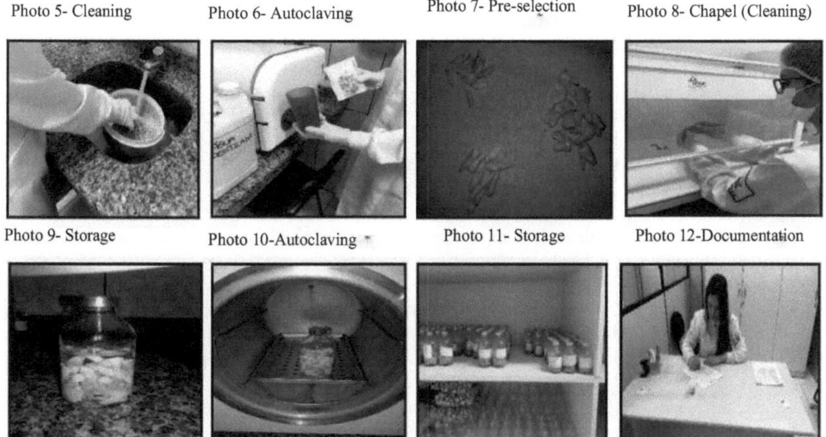

Photo 9- Storage Photo 10-Autoclaving Photo 11- Storage Photo 12-Documentation

Source - the authors.

Therefore, the microbiological analysis showed that the stored specimens were free from contamination by pathogenic microorganisms according to the laboratory reports, with the exception of the control group, which revealed the presence of saprophytic bacteria, which are bacteria that do not develop in living organisms and feed on the waste present in these organisms, i.e. they are non-pathogenic bacteria. They are not harmful to the human body.

For the Knoop microhardness test, the samples were polished, positioned and fixed to the base of the microhardness tester perpendicular to the tip of the load applicator. The hardness measurements were taken using the *Shimadzu®* model *HMV-2- Series - Micro Hardness Tester microhardness tester* (photo 13). On each slice, 1 endentation (photo 14) was performed with a diamond tip attached to the device with 100 grams of force for 5 seconds and in the middle third regions.

Photo 13-Microdurometer Photo 14-Endentaçao

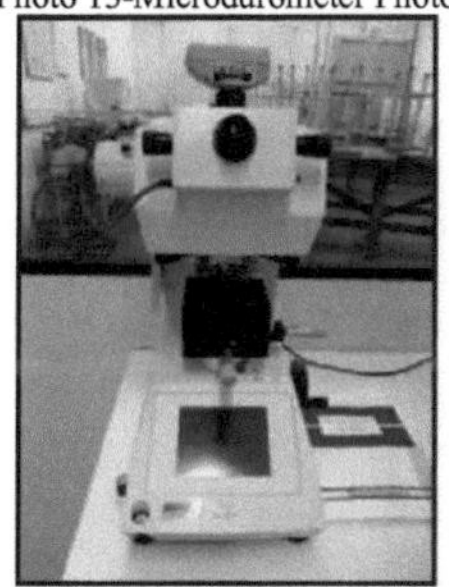 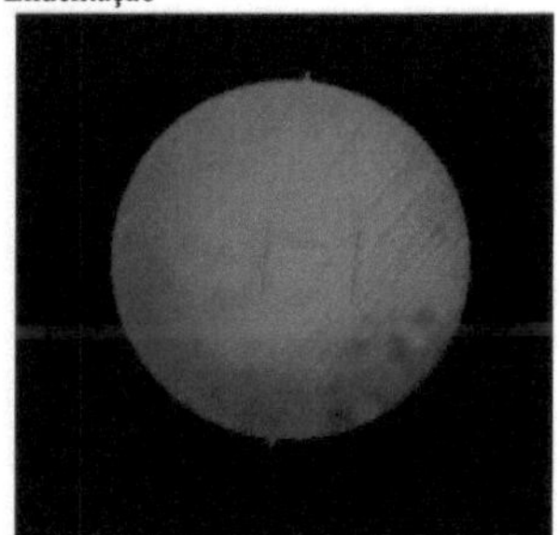

Source: the authors.

Knowledge of the physical and mechanical properties of dental tissue is of great importance. In this way, it is possible to understand and relate the clinical behavior of restorations made with different materials to healthy tooth structure. Among the most important physical and mechanical properties are modulus of elasticity, strength and hardness (MEREDITH et al., 1996; XU et al., 1998; MAHONEY et al., 2000).

The dental enamel microhardness averages found in the tests in this study, using ANOVA analysis, ranged from 233.40 to 69.10, given that several studies on microhardness have shown that dental enamel has higher values than dentin. A statistical difference was found in the samples that were stored and sterilized for 2 years (G5), i.e. the hardness of the teeth decreased significantly. In the control group (G1), in which the samples were cleaned and decontaminated once, the variation in microhardness was between (312 - 163). According to Meredith et al. (1996), the average hardness value for enamel is between 270 and 350 Knoop. However, the standard deviations for these values show wide and significant variations. These variations can be produced by factors such as histological characteristics, chemical composition, sample preparation, as well as loading and reading errors in the indentation length.

In the present study, it can be seen that for microhardness in healthy enamel, the methods analyzed decreased the hardness values. Autoclaving may have altered the microhardness averages due to the heat under pressure generated during the sterilization process, which can lead to the breakdown of ionic bonds between collagen and hydroxyapatite (PARSELL et al., 1998).

The autoclave sterilization process subjects enamel specimens to humid conditions under high temperature and pressure, which may act as the culprit for the changes observed in the elemental chemical composition of the enamel surface (VIANA, 2013). Therefore, we hypothesize that the increase in temperature and high pressure during autoclaving denatures the organic component of enamel, thus affecting microhardness.

In view of the results obtained, it is important to study the methods used to sterilize the dental substrate, as these have an influence on the hardness properties of the tooth.

4 CONCLUSION

From the research carried out, it can be seen that according to the data collected by the microbiological analysis, the dental elements stored in the Human Teeth Biobank at UNOESC Campus .loacaba are free from contamination, so the operational methods adopted are safe, effective and also prolong the useful life of the teeth, eliminate the risk of cross-contamination and reduce the labor required for maintenance.

As for microhardness, it was found that it decreased with increasing storage time, which was statistically significant when comparing the groups with each other, but there is still a need for further studies to identify whether it is storage time or autoclaving that alters microhardness.

STUDY OF THE MICROBIOLOGICAL CONTROL AND MICRODURE OF THE TEETH STORED IN THE HUMAN'S TOOTH BIOBANK OF UNOESC JOACABA

ABSTRACT

The Human's Teeth Biobank (HTB) of the UNOESC Joaçaba, it's a very important space in the University for the Odontology course, because it is a place used to store human's teeth, which should be considered a source of cross contamination, therefore the certain decontamination and store permit the support of the physical properties of the teeth and the decrease the risk of cross contamination. The purpose with the study was to evaluate the quality of the microbiological control of the teeth stored in the HTB, according to their adopted SOP's, the real effectiveness and whether the method doesn't influence the physical characteristics of dental elements such as microhardness. The work was carried out by the in vitro study medium with human teeth in the laboratory of the HTB, stored in distilled H20 and hermetically sealed, using for the tests the microdurometer and the technique of seeding by exhaustion for microbiological analysis. Through the results, it was observed that as samples evaluated if available free of contamination and statiscally, only changes occur in microhardness of teeth stored within two years. It's verified that the dental elements stored in the UNOESC BDH, are free of contamination, and can be used safely in laboratory research activities, and with a relation to microhardness, it was verified that the dental elements that suffered greater variation in physical characteristics were those of the G5, not allowing it to be used in researches related to microhardness. Demonstrating that the stored teeth in the HTB of the UNOESC would be used in the different laboratory research activities.

Key-words: Tooth Biobank. Microbiology. Microhardness. Tooth.

REFERENCES

ARENDS, J; TEN BOSCH, JJ. Demineralization and remineralization evaluation techniques. **Journal Dental Research,** v.71, p.924-928, apr.1992.

BEGOSSO, M; IMPARATO, JCP; DUARTE, D. Current status of the organization of human tooth banks in dental schools in Brazil. **Revísta de Pós- Graduagao,** v.8, n.1, p.23-28, jan-mar. 2001.

BRAUER Delia S. et al. Effect of sterilization by gamma radiation on nano-mechanical properties of teeth. **Dental Materials**, v.24, n.8, p.1137-1140, aug. 2008.

COSTA, Simone de Melo. et al. Human teeth in dental education: origin, use, decontamination and storage by UNIMONTES academics, **ABENO Magazine**, v.7, n.1, p. 6/12,Jan/Apr 2007.

DE-DEUS G; PACIORNIK S; MAURICIO MH. Evaluation ofthe effect ofEDTA, EDTAC and citric acid on the microhardness of root dentine. **International Endodontic Journal**, v.39, n.5, p. 401/407, mai. 2006.

DE-DEUS Gustavo. et al. Longitudinal and quantitative evaluation of dentin demineralization when subjected to EDTA, EDTAC, and citric acid: a co-site digital optical microscopy study. **Oral Surgery Oral Medicine Oral Pathology Oral Radiology**, v.105,n.3, p.391/397, mar. 2008.

FARRET, M. et al. Influence of methodological variables on shear bond strength. **Dental Press Journal of Orthodontics**, v.15,n.1, p. 80/88, jan-feb. 2010.

IMPARATO, Jose Carlos Pettorossi et al. Banco de Dentes Humanos. Editora Maio, Curitiba, 2003.

LEE Jason Jonghyuk. et al. Using extracted teeth for research: the effect of storage medium and sterilization on dentin bond strengths. **The Journal of The American Dental Association**, v.138, n.12, p.1599/1603, dec. 2007.

MAHONEY E. et. al. The hardness and modulus of elasticity of primary molar teeth: an ultramicro-indentation study. **Journal of Dentistry,** v.28, n.8, p. 589/594, nov. 2000.

MEREDITH Neil, et al. Measurement of the microhardness and Young's modulus of human enamel and dentine using an indentation technique. **Archives of Oral Biology**, v.41,n.6, p.539/545, jun. 1996.

MOSCOVICH H. et al. In vitro dentine hardness following gamma-irradiation and freezing. **Journal of Dentistry**, v.27, n.7, p. 503-507, sep. 1999.

NASSIF Alessandra Cristina da Silva. et al. Structure of a Human Tooth Bank. **Pesquisa Odontológica Brasileira**, v.17, n.1, p. 70/74, 2003.

PAGNINO, R. P. et al. Airborne microorganisms collected in a preclinical dental laboratory. **Journal of Dental Education,** v.49, n.9, p. 653/655, set. 1985.

PARSELL, D. E. et al. The effect of steam sterilization on the physical properties and perceived cutting characteristics of extracted teeth. **Journal of Dental Education**, v.62, n.3,p. 260/263, mar. 1998.

PASHLEY David; OKABE Atsuko; PARHAM Phillip. The relationship between dentin microhardness and tubule density. **Dental Traumatology**, v.1, n.5, p. 176/179, Oct. 1985.

PATIL ChetanR; UPPIN Veerendra. Effect of endodontic irrigating solutions on the microhardness and roughness of root canal dentin: an in vitro study. **Indian Journal of Dental Research,** v.22, n.22, p. 22/27, abri. 2011.

SILVA, MF. et al. Influence of the type of storage and method of disinfection of extracted teeth on adhesion to tooth structure. **Revista de Odontologia da Universidade Cidade de Sâo Paulo**, v.18 n.2, p.175-180, May-Aug. 2006.

VIANA Patricia Gabriela Sabino. Influence of different methods of sterilizing dental enamel on its morphology, chemical composition, structure and biofilm formation in vitro. 2013. 133f. **Dissertation (Master's Degree in Dentistry),** Universidade Estadual Paulista, UNESP Araraquara School of Dentistry, Sâo Paulo.

WHITE James M. et al. Sterilization of teeth by gamma radiation. **Journal of Dental Research**, v.73, n.9, p.1560-1567, sep. 1994.

XU HH. et al. Indentation damage and mechanical properties of human enamel and dentin. **Journal of Dental Research,** v.77, n.3,p. 472/480, mar. 1998.

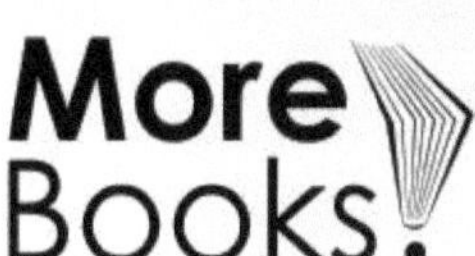

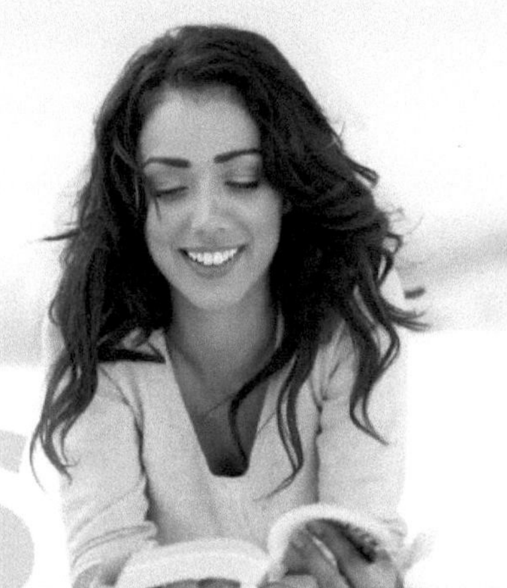

Buy your books fast and straightforward online - at one of world's fastest growing online book stores! Environmentally sound due to Print-on-Demand technologies.

Buy your books online at
www.morebooks.shop

Kaufen Sie Ihre Bücher schnell und unkompliziert online – auf einer der am schnellsten wachsenden Buchhandelsplattformen weltweit! Dank Print-On-Demand umwelt- und ressourcenschonend produziert.

Bücher schneller online kaufen
www.morebooks.shop

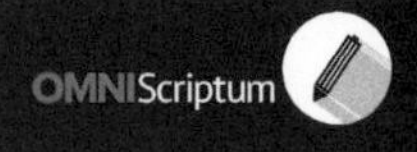

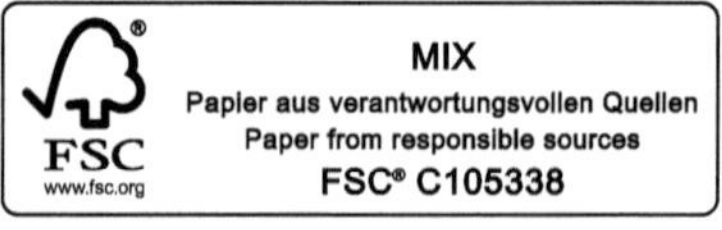

Printed by Books on Demand GmbH, Norderstedt / Germany